# *Tattletales* of a
# SPEECH-LANGUAGE
# PATHOLOGIST

The CFY's Guide To Surviving The Skilled Nursing Facility.

SULEIKA J. PRYCE
M.S., CCC-SLP

Professional review by Elena Borelli, M.S. PAC, BCPA
Editing and book design by Melissa Niemann
Book cover design by Michiel van der Wal

# TABLE OF CONTENTS

# Part One
## ORIENTATION

# 1

# AUTHOR'S NOTE

I am Suleika Jenelle Pryce, M.S., CCC-SLP. Before the letters became an addition to my name, I was just a girl with a church school upbringing and a Brooklyn bite. My humble beginnings led me from the brick-slab patterned East Flatbush to the hills and grasslands of the Blue Mountain in Pennsylvania. Before long, I switched lanes to attend Temple University in the heart of North Philadelphia, one of the top five rough-and-tough American cities. My time at Adelphi University appeared to be a stroll through its colorful urban ecosystem. In reality, life was challenging and no walk in the park. The time spent there came at the apex of a journey of self-seeking, rejection, and nearly endless obstacles. As a result, I was convinced of my ability to survive anywhere by the time I began my clinical fellowship year in August 2018. What I didn't realize was that two years down the road, I would have this story to tell.

If you asked me to count, I would say I've wanted to do no less than one million things with my life. Before I decided on speech-language pathology, I wanted to be a veterinarian, computer technician, and author. After I got my bachelor's degree, I wanted to be a personal trainer, public health advocate, mental health counselor, and an author. After graduating with my Master's, I wanted to travel, do photography, and—of course—become an author.

But how did I know speech pathology was the right career path for me?

Coming from a bilingual family, and having an elder brother who is Deaf, language and the art of communicating has always surrounded me. However, it wasn't interesting. It was just life. Besides, studying health and medicine was a far better use of time than learning about languages. As I got older, the desire to educate and serve the Deaf community catapulted me into this new field that became more interesting the more I learned about it.

Speech pathology is the best thing that has ever happened to me, because apart from learning language and linguistics, it opened doors of opportunity. It simplified and answered mysteries of my life and revealed the world to me in so many ways. The greatest gift that speech pathology has offered me (thus far) is publishing my first book.

One thing I know for sure: it was my destiny to become a writer ever since I could hold a pencil. My introduction to Linguistics flipped my boredom with languages on its head. That's when I realized writing is just another form of language. When I started learning speech pathology, my knowledge of how people inspect and create expectations for language helped shape and develop my writing. Discovering how language changes literally everything, and how I can be a part of such an amazing process still amazes me every day!

Falling in love with dysphagia, well... that's a whole other story.

# 2

# INTRODUCTION

I'll be clear—I entitled this book Tattletales for a reason. With love comes great responsibility. It is mine to use what I've gained to better you, the newest generation of clinicians of speech-language and swallowing, by preparing you for what the skilled nursing facility (SNF) offers. Nothing here is a secret. None of it is protected information. Although this was true before I began my fellowship year, I have to confess: my view of the SNF as a full-time employee differed entirely from my view of it when I was a student. I think this is because as students we develop certain expectations; but, as with so many other aspects of life, reality often offers an unexpected experience. As you'll discover while reading, I have had to learn much of the SNF up close—things that didn't meet the naked eye.

This book is meant to give you an accurate framework of what to expect, help you decide whether a SNF is the best place to start your journey in the field, and inspire you to accept a great position, whether in this setting or elsewhere.

As I was taught in my clinical placements during grad school, it's best to start with the positive. In a SNF, a speech-language pathologist has access to an oak of professionals. They are skilled in a variety of fields of knowledge, readily reachable, and always have an answer. Even better, they help you create a 'whole' view of your patients and share insights to help you better understand the workplace, system, and world around you. Your daily interactions with fellow professionals will help you become a better clinician and person. In this fast-paced and ever-changing setting, you will learn how to manage your time and emotions and make better decisions. Ideally, you will leave your CFY a confident and well-informed clinician.

What you won't be is perfect.

The individuals on your caseload will be ever changing (far more than the facility and its expectations and systems). There is no limit to what you might be challenged with in terms of new and complicated medical diagnoses that may be concomitant with neurogenic or cognitive issues. Your patients will not always follow A-Z procedures; and your ability to communicate effectively, report and refer appropriately, and document everything will remain the most important puzzle piece.

While I have just emphasized a changing environment, I have to contradict myself: some days and weeks may make you feel like a hamster running on a wheel. Doing two handfuls of paperwork in a day, checking in on notes and orders, in-servicing, and doing repetitive caregiver training... well, these are just the reality of the workplace. Not to mention that in long-term care, which typically makes up a greater percentage of the SNF than short-term care, things can get a bit static. My SNF experience has been the greatest test of patience and endurance. I say this to say, Tattletales is not the glitter and gold of working in a SNF.

I wrote this book to reflect on my two-year experience as a speech-language and swallow therapist. I share what has propelled me forward, and what held me back, what surprised me, what has become common and acceptable, and what is downright unavoidable. Regard Tattletales as unmitigated, honest, and transparent storytelling of a speech-language pathology graduate's day-to-day life in a SNF. As in all aspects of life, your story will differ from mine. Although the SNF was not the setting I wished to stay in nearing the end of my CFY, I still hope to reveal my victories and failures in such a way that can help you understand why this experience was so meaningful for me. I also hope to help you learn what's possible, how to manage challenges in the moment, and how you might have to clean up later.

In short: this is your guide to surviving your clinical fellowship year.

# 3

# MIRROR, MIRROR

*A Guide to Yourself*

This is a quick self-review about your goals and what has brought you this far. If possible, write all over this book. Highlight. Staple other useful texts and lists that you find. Notate. Be tangential. Write your own stories. It's your guide to surviving. I'm just your personal Steve Irwin, and I do play with wild animals on and off the clock. (Really—we have a comfort dog named Fluffy.)

I came into the field of speech-language pathology because I wanted to:

_____

_____

_____

As I have pursued this field, my goals and feelings surrounding it have changed in this way:

_____

_____

_____

I would feel like pursuing speech-language pathology  was a waste of time if:

_____

_____

_____

I would feel like pursuing speech-language pathology  was worth it if:

_____

_____

_____

If I were to pursue anything other than speech-language pathology, it would be:

_____

_____

_____

I want to learn more about the following disorders or differences (things that seem to deviate from the norm-but are actually just related to some cultural or linguistic habit):

_____

_____

_____

Because...

_____

_____

_____

Which supervisor, friend or family member, or important person's voice rings in my head when I think of doing this job; and why have they had this influence on me?

_____

_____

_____

Who has most discouraged me on this career path? What did I learn from that?

_____

_____

_____

My most memorable clinical experience or client in grad school was:

_____

_____

_____

A time I had to think on my feet:

_____

_____

_____

How do I respond to things not going my way and being told, "no?"

_____

_____

_____

How do I take care of myself while taking care of those around me?

_____

_____

_____

After writing into each segment (or just considering each question), I want to follow up. Yes, all homework needs to be checked—even if it's self-checked.

- You expected something to come from this particular field and subfield, and you will get it. You just have to learn how. By sharing my journey with you, I hope to give you a head-start in this learning process.

- Your path is not unidirectional. In fact, it's allowed to be as complex as you want it to be. This field allows exactly that. You can love both adults and children, like medical settings as much as you like educational settings, and you can even travel.

- Your CFY can be the most useful year of your career, but it can also be the most useless. It won't make or break you, but why not spend it learning what you really want to?

- That supervisor, parent, friend, or whoever acted as a turning point for you: whether it was through their efforts to encourage or discourage you... Guess what? You're here now. Send them a postcard.

- You must be a clinical writer. Your professors were not exaggerating that part. If school didn't prepare you well enough, I hope I can help.

- Learning to be culturally sensitive is a part of ethically conducting our practice. Thinking of what makes you, you, helps you determine how to relate to others. There is no general list waiting around anywhere online or even in this book about every nationality and cultural identifier and what to expect. The only answer is being exactly who you need to be to you first. That way, you will be prepared to interact with people like and unlike you.

- Your best and worst character traits will show up on the job. Enhance the good ones and by golly, work on the bad ones! Don't find yourself years down the line with the same bad habits.

- You will find yourself in situations that require quick thinking. In fact, you will find yourself in situations you cannot even handle. You are not alone, but you hold a very important place in the process. If you can learn to push through, you will be better for doing so.

- Nothing on this planet is perfect. I would even say the universe almost strives to prove to us that we do not have the last say. So, it's important to take another look within, think creatively, be a solution-maker, and make the absolute best of every minute—billable or non-billable.

- The speech pathologist is only one part of who you are. If you're being 80% productive, the other 20% still counts on you to be attentive to self-care, eating breakfast AND lunch, and drowning yourself in paperwork and continuing education only if you promise yourself an aloe and essential oil bath after.

If this was at all meaningful or motivating, you are ready for the rest of this book and the rest of your career. Thank you for attending my TED Talk. Now, let's get into it.

# 4

# INTENT

*A Guide to Landing the Job*

When you're looking for companies to apply to, it's important to talk to your mentors, professors, and peers about it. You never know who you know. That being said, you don't have to jump at the first opportunity that rears its head. Intent is the first step. Heedfulness and conscientiousness in your pursuit of the field will be evident to future employers. Whatever your area of interest, ensure that you have an attractive resume that highlights how much effort you have put into gaining exposure and experience in it. Then there is diligence. To me, this means staying true to what you want while staying true to who you are. Bring more than just paper facts to an interview—bring you. My motto is: the resume gets the interview, but you get the job. Remember that, apart from spending six or seven years in school for this moment, you have shed blood and tears along the way to make it through tough clinical placements. At this point of your journey, you know where your focus needs to be and what you aren't willing to go without. The CFY is truly not any more difficult than what you've already been through. What you want to be most sure of is that it is useful for, and caters to, the SLP you want to become.

I would say the greatest help to landing the job I wanted was how long I had spent knowing I wanted to do it. Now, it wasn't my dream job. In fact, I had seen the inside of nursing facilities before, and damn near screamed in terror of it all. I wanted the job, though, because it was an amazing opportunity to work with an adult population in a medical setting that wasn't a hospital. As a student, I came to think of hospitals as a little too busy and impersonal, even though I had a great rapport with the patients I treated.

I knew I didn't want to be in a school, because the thought of being in the school setting made me feel too much like a teacher and less like a health professional. Group therapy was outside of my comfort zone, so when they started encouraging it in the SNF, I had unexplainable, immense chills. Well, go figure: it is more profitable to provide more therapy in less time. After all, it's not that bad.

I still feel the same about the school setting; but during holidays and winter and summer breaks, I am so jealous of my peers in the Department of Education.

I knew early intervention was on my checklist, but I didn't think it was something I needed to learn under strong supervision. To be brutally honest, I wanted to pick the hardest thing I could do as a speech-language pathology clinical fellow to make sure I could do it properly by the end of ten months. I would say I compared it to learning to drive in New York City. If you can master that, everywhere else is a breeze. Trust me.

Every other area I looked into was either so exclusive I didn't qualify, or it was too boring. I thought the SNF was a pleasant middle ground where I could learn everything.

I was almost right!

I knew what I didn't want to do—or what I didn't want to do yet, at least. Maybe my points of view differ from yours; maybe they're too simple, or maybe they're completely wrong. I don't know. All I can say is that it helped me to narrow down and choose a small company that I liked which offered the opportunity for a good starting salary at $64,000 gross annual pay, opportunities all over New York City and upstate, with strong potential for growth, paid time off, and direct access to the company leaders. They were patient and attentive to their employees and actively involved and ready to teach. I didn't know all of that at the beginning, but something about when you know... YOU REALLY KNOW! Find the job you want.

Here's where I sort of felt I didn't have the control: when I applied to my company, they hired me on the spot in January. Unfortunately, I didn't start my position until the end of August. OUCH. It was life as usual—until I graduated in May. After that, I became terrified that things would not go my way anymore. I was pulling coins from deep in the couch cushions and selling water bottles on the busy streets of Brooklyn.

I was broke, broke...

Another thing I didn't have control over, while dealing with an agency, was the type of facility I'd end up in. I didn't know the difference between long-term, short-term, sub-acute, outpatient care, or assisted living. I went with what I got, because I didn't know what I was in for, and every other company that contracted with medical settings in New York City told me, "No". If I knew anything, it was that I didn't want to move to some small, snowy town in the middle of New York State, where jobs seemed to be much more plentiful.

While moving upstate was something I'd originally considered happily, taking a visit there was less than motivating for me. This was in most part because I felt absolutely unrepresented in the demographics, and it made me uncomfortable. I'm not talking about age. In fact, being young and working with older people is rewarding for several reasons. What I really mean is that there aren't too many black or brown people on those sides. It really crossed the line when there weren't any Giants fans in Utica, NY! Jokes aside, I knew I wanted to be in New York City—my home, my place, my melting pot. Even if it meant my only other choice would be to work with preschool children, I would take it instead. I can never be happy in a place where the norm doesn't speak to my cultural spirit. That's what I meant when I said you should be true to who you are in your pursuit of finding a job. Remember that an enormous chunk of your life will revolve around work, so being happy in it is important.

To be clear, my workplace was largely represented by the Caribbean and Latin communities. Known for their raw and creative linguistic natures, they can turn a regular gray workplace into a colorful comedy scene in seconds. Regular, annoying workplace procedures are the headline of our version of Whose Line Is It Anyway? As for the people from the lower Americas, for whom everything becomes conversation and 'dramatic' is mainstream, it truly can be a grave tragedy when the kitchen hasn't cooked their curry correctly, an in-service makes it past the hour-long limit, or the entire building is regulating extreme temperatures during the winter or summer months without properly functioning air conditioning equipment. The response of the general public—staff and patients included—can make the day go twice as fast or twice as slow. Anyway, it's what makes me feel like I stand a chance at connecting naturally to my atmosphere, even if it means sometimes struggling through my self-taught Spanish and all of my gestural languages to provide non-English speaking patients some level of quality care.

Getting the job can be quick, but you never quite know what to expect when working through an agency. The time it took to finalize my actual position was outrageous. The agency and facility were completely new to one another, making the turnover of rehab professionals a tad bit more complicated. Everything seemed to be in free fall; the agency tried to send me to Yonkers, at least an hour from where I lived. Thus I waited, faithfully. At the end of an interesting summer, I received a location that was comfortable and a reasonable distance from my house. The parking sucked, but I realized I wouldn't win every battle.

My best advice: prepare yourself for some downtime after graduating. Your company may promise you an immediate start, but it never hurts to have a backup plan.

# Part Two
## WELCOME TO THE SNF

# 5

# THE NEW GUY ON THE BLOCK

## *A Guide to Starting Off on the Right Foot*

Your first few days—weeks, maybe—might present you with experiences of people looking right through you. That may be an indicator that the turnover in your SNF setting is high. At least, that was it for me. From rehab staff, to the kitchen staff, to the patients you serve, new faces are not uncommon. Fear not.

In this chapter, I want to help you learn how to start things off right. Keeping in mind that the SNF is not just a work office, but a thriving community, it's important to remember that you are an active and positive member of it.

### HELLO, MY NAME IS...

Establish yourself strongly. Say your name and explain what you do to staff, patients, and their families. It's a respectful gesture that not only offers a start to a solid rapport, but can strongly affect how people view you and take in what you say. If you inquire enough, you get to know the people around you as well. Nine times out of ten, they will help you do your job better.

We'll dig deeper into this in the next chapter, called Friend or Foe.

After two years, people I worked with knew my face, my title, or my name. Usually, it wasn't all three. TWO YEARS. It's far from rare to hear a page over the intercom: "Speech Therapist, please call extension...!" It doesn't bother me that people don't always remember my given name, or that half the time they approach me, it's for something that is someone else's job. I've been toting an uncommon name for 27 years, so nothing new there. It took me aback for a bit, though, that people were regularly asking me for wheelchairs for new admissions. Often, in the same hour I tried to bill for speech therapy, I was mistaken for a social worker, nurse, and physical therapist!

You'll discover that our scope is often and severely misinterpreted, even after people get to know your face. Don't let this get to you. Personally, it gave me joy to gently remind people what the heck my role in the SNF really entailed. As I did that, I gladly accepted the opportunity to redirect them to the right professional for their needs, but encouraged them to return to me if a patient was coughing during meals, or if they noticed a patient developing a new cognitive issue, like sudden confusion.

## THE GOOD SAMARITAN

You do want to put yourself in others' shoes, sometimes. Good Samaritans are far and few between, but people around you notice these tiny acts of justice. Besides, don't they just feel good? This applies to staff and residents—even those who aren't on your schedule. We work with vulnerable people, most of whom really just need a 'somebody.' They tend to forget often, but many of them can still identify you as the nice kid who grabbed them a glass of water, tied their shoelaces, or adjusted their chair so they could see the television better. And, yes, they will ask again. An opportunity to have small talk and do kind things for the elderly is nothing to turn aside.

Consider co-workers who may feel overwhelmed, short of hands, or short of time. If possible and ethical, don't hesitate to help others with their tasks. For me, just because it didn't necessarily fit into my job description or my tasks for the day, it didn't mean I had no time for it. Two minutes spent helping to transfer a patient, or turning a dysphagia session into feeding my patient lunch, did not take much away from me. Try to be mindful and kind as you begin your journey. At times, you may feel more concerned about your productivity percentage. Being helpful is not only productive, but immensely rewarding as it makes you an active part of your little community.

## COMMUNICATION

Go with a mindset ready to learn, rather than to instruct... Ask more questions! This can be just to get a foot in the water to test the people you'll be working with. Know a little bit about what workplace values are. You don't have to learn everything about your co-workers, but it doesn't hurt one bit to at least relate to them in some way or to have a name or two you can call. Test their levels of responsiveness to you, and perhaps they can help you establish a good working presence in the facility.

Your new job may come with a set of procedures and guidelines you weren't exposed to as a student. Ideally, you'd spend a few weeks in training to learn about these. Or maybe, instead, a stork will just drop you head-first into a several-hundred-bed box without windows, a lot of squeaky doors, paper charts, and slow elevators.

Don't panic!

Perhaps there's something you can't find, or something you don't understand. Just ask. Most people will respond, even if their eyes never turn in your direction and their computer keyboard continues to sound off from quick finger strikes. You'll get this a lot. It reflects how busy people are in the SNF setting, but not how attentive they are. Fifty percent of the time, you might get an, "I don't know," the first time you ask a question to someone who really should know. Don't take it personally. The best thing you can follow up with is, "who might know?" Worse comes to worst, you have your supervisor and rehab director to clarify the simplest to the most complicated issues you may come across.

Perhaps there's something you think another staff is unintentionally doing wrong, or you think a system is just not working the way it's supposed to. If you're anything like me, you'll have a push-and-pull with yourself to find the middle ground of not keeping completely still, but also not exerting a heavy hand to tip people's noses. Knowing the what, why, and the then what? may set you up for a better and necessary discourse.

Certainly, you are educated to apply what you know. When you're new, you might find that something is not the way it should be. You could think that maybe you should play it cool and see what happens. I say, not at all—what you saw will happen again. There's not enough healthy change in SNFs, and I wouldn't look forward to witnessing the sporadic improvement or resolve of an issue overnight. You should explain as early as possible why you think something is important to attend to. Your recommendations have a basis and are reasonable. If your ideal is to change an aspect of the way staff or the facility carries out something, I encourage you to address the issue. You should especially apply pressure if one or several patients are at risk or being underserved.

If your CFY supervisor is not in the same building, make an effort to keep him or her abreast of everything you notice and ask for advice. Many a time, my supervisor accompanied me to meetings with administrators and got me on track for in-servicing. I was very thankful for that kind of support. It isn't your place to facilitate big changes without leadership, anyway. The clinical fellowship year is for learning with a guide, so use your time there to do just that.

Learning the importance of communication, for a communication science specialist, may seem redundant. Well, I'll say this: with communication, this job is hard. Without communication, this job is hell. You communicate not only to get your point across but also to not become mechanical. Being programmed to the will and way of everyone else, or to regurgitate the same actions and information repeatedly, will rob you of the very joy you can experience in a place like this.

I speak first-hand when I say it's tempting to fall into that trap in this position.

The next chapters will dive into the living body of communication—the lasting impressions you can make on your patients and your team of professionals.

Being the 'new guy on the block,' you may believe that the impression you make on others will be rather insignificant. However, how you conduct yourself and what you choose to do in various situations is not inconsequential. Respect begets respect, and it carries over. Who you prove to be over time, especially with obstacles thrown onto your path, will be duly noted by your co-workers, directors, and residents.

# 6

# FRIEND OR FOE?

## A Guide to Your Co-workers

While going about your daily activities on the job, you'll get to know who's who, what they do, and why you need them. No one is truly your foe—we are all in this together. Know that being in a SNF, there are a lot of intelligent people who are differently inclined. Managing your workspace in a way that makes you comfortable, respected, and resourceful is key.

That being said, some of your job tasks may come with a push back. Depending on the general layout and organization of your facility, you may run into instances where your toes get stepped on, or worse. Confident communication is an effective method of resolution in most cases, and may totally avoid uncomfortable run-ins.

The following is a run-down of the people you will work with regularly.

### YOUR REHAB DIRECTOR

This will be your boss—someone you will get to know quickly. While you may have distant supervision from a licensed speech-language pathologist, this person is always at your workplace and can oversee and help you manage your workload. Rehab directors are dedicated to their jobs, and a lot is expected of them. Considering that rehab is usually agency-based rather than facility-based, they are the faces of the agency. They know about insurance, agency money, facility money, family planning, and a whole lot more. They make your schedules and are the starting and ending point of your therapeutic plan. Rehab directors are not typically professionals in the field of speech pathology. Instead, they will more likely be occupational or physical therapists, and they are normally open to our clinical judgment, as long as we are confident about it.

In tangent, I've seen rehab directors come and go; each story was unique. Though this was the case for me, it's not a typical thing—rehab directors normally stay put for years. My directors handled the work so differently. With their influence, they truly have the power to set the tone of the department and answer the question: how effective are we as a team? When rehab directors change, the expectations of you as a service provider change slightly, too. This may be evident in the new director's increased or decreased attention to your productivity. Perhaps you may find that you have more meetings worked into your schedule to create more opportunities to be active in care planning, or in whatever he or she deems to be beneficial to you, the department, and the patient.

A rehab director's authority style becomes apparent during conflict resolution. I've been generally blessed to have had directors who defended me, spoke on my behalf, and believed in my abilities and work ethic. You need someone with a positive energy that recognizes your worth and accommodates the various needs you may have. In a rehab world in which speech-language pathologists hardly fit in with the occupational therapists (OTs) and physical therapists (PTs), inclusion, support, and staying in the know is truly the grit of what a rehab director offers at both a personal and professional level.

The rating on the rehab director: friend.

Remember that, although the rehab director will generally support you and truly is a friend, he or she works under immense pressure. Their urgency for picking up more and more patients may sometimes come over as them not being as considerate of what you or the patient can handle. Rehab mostly acts as the money launderer of the facility. In many ways, rehab keeps the short- and long-term wheels running by identifying cases that can be useful for the facility's monetary goals. Sometimes pressure may result from that and, in turn, affect your caseload in good and bad ways. While I've never perceived a director as being mean or aggressive about this, I have felt that they could be pushy. Having a thick skin, the ability not to take things personally, and being able to communicate effectively are important skills to develop, because you may find yourself in the position of needing to reiterate your personal and professional ethics to evade this type of pressure.

## DIETICIANS

You'll spend a great deal of your time communicating with the dieticians at the SNF. They should be the first—aside from yourself—to know that a diet or liquid consistency has been changed. If your situation is like mine, you'll have their cell numbers or extensions within reach at all times. They act as your point of communication with the kitchen, your source of information about percutaneous endoscopic gastrostomy (PEG) tube feeding and weight management, and act as the overseers who make sure sugar, sodium, and fluid limitations are fitting for each patient. They are also, fortunately, the people you can spend the most time talking with about your patients' food. Your peers in the rehab gym will tolerate about three sentences about this—it's just not their thing.

While interactions with the dietician can be informative and helpful, it can also be a bit of a push-and-pull when people from different fields have to settle on a decision regarding a particular patient. For instance, what looks great from a rehab standpoint, may not be as great from a dietary standpoint. Let's say a patient loves fried finger foods. From our standpoint, the patient can tolerate it, is happy, and not at risk of failure to thrive. From the dietician's standpoint, however, the patient would only benefit from a low-fat and low-sodium diet to manage obesity and heart disease—aspects that we speech-language pathologists rarely consider. Maybe the compensatory strategy we come up with is to alternate solids and liquids frequently, but the dietician has implied a fluid restriction. Maybe the dietician is comfortable with the PEG tube being the only means of nutrition and hydration, but we are trained to wean aggressively. The helpfulness of effective communication skills come in best in such cases. As you learn what other professionals do, the ability to anticipate some of these run-ins becomes easier.

The rating on the dietician: friend.

For me, it has also been possible to see my dietician as my non-SLP, SNF advisor. While they don't have the same knowledge of dysphagia that we use to treat our patients, they study things like the International Dysphagia Diet Standardization Initiative (IDDSI) and have age-old legends about diet consistencies gone wrong.

Once, twice, or more times, this dynamic has led to dieticians stepping on my toes, making decisions without notifying me or even consulting with me. I've been told I wasn't 'essential' when a dysphagia patient lost dentures, or when family members wanted an immediate response to a new behavior from a patient. With the dieticians a step ahead of me on the building's communication hierarchy, I could only stay calm, screen, and document.

## KITCHEN STAFF

The kitchen is the busiest place in a nursing home. It isn't at every facility that you will be in direct contact with the kitchen staff; however, you need to know how to get what you need for your daily therapy. Between my facilities, I always found that the quickest and most efficient way to secure my need for food items was to head straight to the kitchen. Some other therapists prefer to call and have a staff member deliver a food item at their convenience. It's for certain that the farther in advance the speech-language pathologist can decide and communicate what they need, the easier everyone's lives are. Generally, I used to be at my busiest during lunch hours. The kitchen staff knew from as early as 10:00 in the morning, for a 12:00 lunch, exactly what I expected for my mealtime rounds. In a SNF, requests can be delivered to the floors at an earlier time with the appropriate notice, as well.

It helps to make a few friends in the kitchen. I used to greet, chat, and joke with the kitchen staff. They were the people most willing to help me out, even if I forgot to call in advance. Coming up with a recurring system is best and allows everyone to achieve the greatest productivity at their jobs.

The rating on kitchen staff: foe.

Perhaps the reason I choose 'foe' is not generalizable to most facilities outside of the ones in which I worked. To put it simply, the kitchen staff know food. Culinary expertise doesn't typically equate to healthy and sound. While the dieticians know food consistencies well, they are unfortunately not in charge of the kitchen, though they are in constant communication with its leaders. The kitchen staff may know some of the patients—in our facility, they held regular meetings for residents to voice their concerns, and the menu was always at the forefront of those discussions. For such occasions and other passing moments over time, the kitchen leaders get to be present and partake in getting to know the people they feed. Otherwise, patients are generally just a code: rack, stack, and ship out for delivery. Sometimes the staff don't get the code right—just like every machine glitches sometimes. The kitchen has often ruined my productivity by glitching on our schedule or giving a patient the wrong consistency. Even more often, I have had experiences where the kitchen leaders gave me hell for no identifiable reason. Further, any menu will have items that cause confusion and even make you worried when it comes to consistency. If you find your patient has a huge ham hero, while their diet orders are for a chopped diet consistency, there's nothing you can do but watch and wait. Hey, potential diet upgrade?

## NURSES

Staff nurses, usually licensed practical nurses or registered nurses, provide day-to-day care for patients. They require skilled knowledge of medicine, wound dressing, tube feeding, and much more. Also, they're the ones who respond first to changes in patients' vital signs and report it to the charge nurse or nursing supervisor, and they report on anything that seems off the mark.

Nursing supervisors differ from one facility to the next in terms of what they do in relation to the speech therapist. I noticed that the nursing supervisors at my primary facility were much more involved and personable. At other facilities I covered, including my secondary facility, communication was much more cut and dried. At the facilities I worked in, morning (7 AM to 3 PM) supervisors were more plentiful and available than evening (3 PM to 11 PM) supervisors. I wouldn't suggest approaching the evening nursing supervisor for anything less than an emergency. At least at my two facilities, they were the only supervisors during their shifts. Keep in mind that they're responsible for every bed—they are busy. You probably won't receive your requests very happily during an evening shift, so tread lightly.

The rating on nurses: friend.

Nurses hold a bad reputation for their bedside manners and responses to other staff. If you know a nurse, you'll agree that they're really angels—angels that talk fast, move quickly, and are unafraid to tell you exactly like it is when you're wrong. Nursing supervisors, especially, don't always wear a big grin, and they don't 'hee-haw' the day away. But that doesn't mean they are unhappy. Understand that their workload is likely immensely stressful every day. They may not be as up-close-and-personal to listen to all of their patients' stories, but they know them by name, number, weight, date, and in all the ways that matter to their sustained life. They make difficult calls, are immediate links to doctors, and approve your orders and consult you when a patient needs you.

## CERTIFIED NURSING ASSISTANTS (CNAS)

The CNA is the most involved person in the patient's day-to-day needs. Honestly, nothing could be done without them. All day long, they clean, wash, feed, transfer, and watch patients. They carry over nursing rehab programs by walking with their wheelchair-bound patients and are quickly called to assist in other departments of the facility if need be. They record important information that nurses and other staff need to know about patients, such as their weight and daily activities. While we are the joints and the nurses and doctors are the bones, CNAs are the meat of the system.

Some CNAs love their jobs, and it shows. These people are quick to jump when a patient needs something; and getting to know their residents is one of the pleasurable parts of the job. Others, who do not love or appreciate their roles, are slower to move, may neglect residents' wants and needs, and are very rarely receptive to new ideas and instruction. They entertain themselves at work by watching television, talking on the phone, gossiping, and complaining about the work they signed up to do.

No matter where along the above mentioned spectrum you may find a CNA on any given day, it's important to maintain a good rapport. It's a necessary part of every day to communicate with them to understand your patients and provide better care for them.

The rating on CNAs: foe.

Sadly, those who are poor listeners far outweigh the ones that are great at it. If you rely on a CNA to carry out your recommendations, you will often need to reiterate and follow up. Because they do not have direct access to orders and care plans, verbal communication and training is a necessity.

## ACTIVITIES STAFF

Activities staff members handle patients' daily access to entertainment, exercise, and learning. They carefully organize the common spaces, decorate and lead activities for holidays, and schedule regular games and trivia to keep the residents alert and happy.

Given a patient with a communication deficit, activities on the floor or general space may take a workload off of your back. They'll bring all the materials, while you just have to guide.

The rating on activities staff: friend.

## REHAB STAFF

Of course, the people with whom you share office space and patients—i.e., rehab staff—are important people with whom you should have a working relationship. As a speech-language pathologist, you'll find some aspects about your patients that will require you to report to or consult with other rehab staff. This will include level of participation, diet intake (which will yield more information about why they have no energy during therapy times), and if the patient needs to rehydrate during therapy and is on an altered or thickened diet. You can also get to an understanding of where the patient is making progress or becoming stagnant. This is key to serving the whole patient and not just your piece of the puzzle.

The rating on rehab staff: friend.

## ADMISSIONS PERSONNEL AND SOCIAL WORKERS

The admissions personnel know everything about assigned beds, expected arrivals, recent arrivals, and transfers. Social workers' and admission personnels' tasks may overlap sometimes.

The social workers are especially helpful in the areas of case management, so if there is an imbalance in the patient's care, or if a patient or family member feels dissatisfied with the care the patient is receiving, the social worker is the person to go to. They prepare the meetings that take place to discuss a patient's care plan, manage where and how the patient will continue on from the completion of their rehab program, and can answer a lot of questions regarding your patient's needs and abilities. They are truly superheroes without capes.

The rating on admission personnel and social workers: friend.

## DIRECTOR OF NURSING SERVICES

The DNS, better known as the director of nursing services, is a high point on the totem pole. Planning, managing, in-servicing, and conflict-resolution are amongst their major responsibilities. The DNS will also take the lead in the human resource management of nursing staff, recruiting, and the hiring and firing processes. When you need to 'apply pressure,' she's the one you report to. She creates and updates policies on precautionary behavior and safety standards based on her knowledge of medicine, health, and wellness.

The rating on the DNS: friend.

## ADMINISTRATOR

The administrator is the 'big man' on campus, only second to the CEO. He is someone that thoroughly understands the dynamics of the SNF. Where the DNS creates policies from a medical standpoint, he is the business-minded driver and enforcer of those policies.

The rating on the administrator: friend.

## PHYSICIAN'S ASSISTANT

The physician's assistant is the doctor's right hand. Sometimes a nurse practitioner, instead of a physician assistant, will fill this role. They are skilled and experienced in all areas of geriatric patients and will coordinate the special physical and cognitive care of patients. These professionals are within closer reach than the physician, who is usually a call (or two) away, rather than just a few steps.

The rating on the physician's assistant: friend.

## THE PHYSICIAN

The hands working in the background, the center of all the decision-making, sign-offs, and check-ins—the physicians—provide care for people at your facility and, in addition, to people in a hospital near your facility. If you can imagine the amount of people that rely on one individual with an MD following his or her name, you can understand how cramped they are for time and attention. While the nursing supervisor can generally handle the simple stuff on your behalf, it is never without the physician's consent. In complex situations, you will call them directly for referrals to other specialized medical professionals for objective tests, important discussions, and for permissions regarding your patients' care. You won't see them in person often—some you'll probably see only once a week.

The rating on physicians: a tie!

I have to say this: a general physician doesn't base his or her decisions on a specific field or background. We, as speech-language pathologists, think differently than the dieticians would for a diet-related issue. As I'd outlined before, it can lead to a crossroads in an extreme situation. The general physician, however, is concerned with the patient's ability to sustain life with fewer complications. Only in rare situations do you find that a physician is notably concerned with a patient's quality of life outside the scope of reducing pain and breathing on their own. However, our view of 'quality' goes into an entirely different realm. In some cases, we have hopes more colorful than the rainbow. The physician may act as a reality checkpoint that you're doing way too much.

My experience with the physicians in my building have ranged from extremely positive to extremely negative. It's to utter misunderstanding and grief when you've done all that you've done to get to where you are now, and be of such little value to someone that holds so much power in this kind of dynamic. It's a grim way to look at the situation, but this is coming from someone who has had recommendations torn to utter shreds by a doctor before. It didn't help that a certain physician had the personality of a cactus, and was willing to publicly berate and yell at me. I don't recall my job contract mentioning anything about a medical bootcamp, but at that moment, I felt like a recruit facing my sergeant at basic training. It never helps that you're new to your field, and someone who's been doing what they do for a long time will be unlikely to exchange what they know for what you know. There are rough points, and while I met my toughest blood-boiling point with a straight face and follow-up of a simple, "Yes, Doctor," I promise that what they have to offer to your professional experience isn't all bad.

## YOUR CLINICAL FELLOWSHIP SUPERVISOR

Last but not least, your clinical fellowship supervisor is the first and most important person you will meet on this journey. He or she will be a speech-language pathologist with few to many more years of experience than you. He or she will be a fountain of knowledge and direction, from up close or from afar. A good clinical supervisor can orient you to the day-in-and-day-out procedures of your job and will walk you through several cases to start you off on the right foot. Ideally, this person will remain available for questions and advice throughout the week. This person, who is an expert with the jargon and therapeutic methods we will discuss later, will review your documentation. They will seek every opportunity to uplift you through constructive criticism and positive feedback.

The rating on the clinical fellowship supervisor is not only friend. This person is family, church, and state.

There are individuals who are not good clinical fellowship supervisors. They might not review your cases and your documentation with fresh eyes; and many times, this is due to them having just as big a caseload as yours, on top of the responsibility for all the additional help you may need. This is the unfortunate cause of many unhappy CFYs. If your clinical supervisor is not your friend, I think you need a new one, effective immediately. When you aren't doing well, he or she should feel as though they aren't doing well, either. This isn't to decrease the value of self-sufficiency and personal motivation—these are 100% necessary to make it over any obstacle you'll read about here. It is, however, to highlight what an enormous waste poor leadership is after you have worked so hard to get to this point.

So, who are we to the rest of the building? This may sound biased biased, but I try my best to be a friend.

In a fleet of professionals in the nursing home setting, I believe the speech-language pathologist is the most personally involved with patients.

Hear me out!

We are the ones who most often see our patients one-on-one, which means our caseloads are fairly small and therefore more personal when compared to OTs and PTs. We are not only trained to listen to their stories for their language and cognitive rehabilitation; we also have the benefit of time to counsel and seek solutions to problems they may have. Unlike other professionals, we are in the unique position to notice subtle things. I like to think that we are their voice to other professionals. Their happiness and safety is also our responsibility (a very hard balance to meet). All that aside, we give them food, and there's no greater love than that.

On a darker note, we are also prominent figures at the end-of-life aspect, which I'll expand on in chapter 16, called Mom and Pop. We honestly don't get enough credit for that. We also don't get enough credit for being the 'social butterfly' of the facility. You'll quickly learn just how many relationships we build around our workplaces in order to get through the day. We don't supervise just one floor. We don't care for just 5 patients on our assignment. We don't just care about how patients enter and leave the building. Instead, we carry the patient and all the people that care for them for the duration of their stay, even if it's from a distance. We're the ones who carry the knowledge of hundreds of individuals: we know their names and faces, where they live, their primary diagnoses, the last time they were hospitalized, and what they eat and why—off the top of the noggin! It's a superpower, really, and it also allows us to respond to patients' needs more efficiently whenever they approach us for help.

We don't get enough credit, my friends.

We tend to bend our backs to make others' jobs easier. We humbly schedule around everyone else and their time with patients (OTs and PTs will definitely steal your patients occasionally), we suck up to dieticians and kitchen staff to get our patients their rightful plates—with snacks!—and we take three patients off CNAs' hands to feed them during meal time. There is no reward but the happiness of your patients. That is why you show up. That is why you push through. That is the reason for everything you do. So, if no one says thank you, just know: I see you.

# 7

# CAPITAL P

*A Guide to People and Power*

Growing up, I was always playfully teased for my name. It never bothered me; in fact, it was always laughable that it seemed so great a difficulty for people to handle my first name in pronunciation and spelling. If only I had a nickel for every time I got a "Shaleika," "Suleekah," "Sri Lanka,"—or something along the lines of wrong. Even more memorable was how people used my last name, Pryce, to satisfy common phrases. In middle school, they regularly referred to me as The Pryce is Right!

Though a complete accident in the naming game, I came to learn that both of mine came with powerful, positive meanings. I appreciated them more because of this. Suleika: a brilliant and beautiful woman with a minor planet named after her in orbit around the sun. Then, contrary to the use of Pryce in reference to "The Price is Right," I learned that Pryce has nothing to do with an amount of money. Instead, it represents enthusiasm.

Despite how fitting I felt these were for me, I found it even more laughable to offset the teasing about my names by adopting a new one: Capital P.

It's going to sound a little silly, but I believe in the nuances of letters, shapes, and numbers just as much as I appreciate the meaning behind a name. To me, they represent something bigger than what they are. It's the same as why people think the number 7 is lucky. I think "p," which inevitably reminds me of the words 'power,' 'pride,' 'patience,' and 'professional,' has got a ring to it, no matter what you put it next to.

Capital P—as an epithet—is a reference to someone of great importance, whom others respect or even fear. We can say 'Pimp' or 'Pimpin' are synonymous to bring greater clarity. Everybody wants to be Capital P. Capital P in the streets, or Capital P on the timesheets...

Alternative to the unethical, immoral, crazed criminal that's sometimes associated with those words, on the job, Capital P is someone making big achievements and lots of money, and being a boss.

For more than a few reasons, this character is admirable. However, for many more reasons, he's not really so realistic for most whose last names aren't Bezos or don't have the alter ego of Tony Stark. You must consider that people living so lavishly don't need to be Capital P in a SNF, because they're already Capital C-E-O. But you also don't have to be a billionaire or receive a big check to obtain or abuse power. In this chapter, I'll elaborate on concepts of power and where it really lies within this setting.

It's probably not something you'll think about right at the start, but here's why it is important: the decision-making dynamics within your working environment include you, both as someone giving their perspective and recommendations, and someone reaping the effects of the decisions of leadership around you. The points I present will hopefully help you evaluate your relationship with and understanding of power, and to apply it objectively as needed in your position.

## THE SYSTEM

First, I have to bring attention to the kind of system we work in. Charles McConnell refers to a scale of a view of organizations based on how they do the things they do[1]. In the job organization system—also known as the 'vertical view'—things are highly procedural. Capital P would appear to be the boss, supervisor, whoever runs things around the place. Regular employees follow directions and create a product. He compares this to manufacturing plants and factories.

I think about pyramid-structured organizations, in which the bottom levels vie to reach closer and closer to the top. The motivation is the money—that's just material. However, the power and freedom that comes into existence is also well-met. There is a promise whispered in your ear that you'll transition into a more passive way of living as you climb higher. If you think about it realistically, it's more like adding cushion to the bottom.

The SNF—and healthcare as a whole—is very distinct. There is a power structure and chain-of-command, like any other functioning organization. But obtaining and using power is much more complicated than climbing a ladder.

> "What makes these differing organizational systems work? Likert contends that the job organization system depends largely on economic motives to keep the wheels turning. That is, everything is so controlled that the only remaining requirement is for people to perform the prescribed steps. Therefore, what keeps the wheels turning are the people who show up for work primarily because they are paid to do so. These people are not expected to exhibit a great deal of judgment; they need only follow instructions.

In the cooperative motivation system, however, there are no rigid controls on activities. Jobs cannot be defined down to the last detail, activities and outputs cannot be accurately predicted or scheduled, and the nature of the work coming into the system cannot be depended upon to conform to a formula. In the cooperative motivation system it is not sufficient that employees simply show up because they are being paid. This system depends to a much larger extent on individual enthusiasm and motivation to keep the wheels turning."[1]

The Effective Health Care Supervisor 6th Ed., Chapter 2
Charles McConnell, 2007

We work in what is, as the above excerpt describes, the cooperative motivation—or a 'horizontal'—system. In a 'vertical' system, where the product is tangible, "that's not my job" is usually a reasonable rebuttal. Everyone's responsibilities are clearly defined and shouldn't overlap or sway much. In the SNF, there is a strong need to do more than just your job.

When it comes to the nitty gritty, we all have a dirty job to do.

## WHAT WE MANAGE

At this stage, you should know that this system depends on the way you think. People technically count on you to say "yes" and "no" and whether to move left or right. In this type of setting, we are catalysts for patients' quality of life. As it is a huge responsibility, it may seem that the way to follow through is to enforce, enforce, enforce, but it is important to know at which points you should take the wheel, and at which you're better off taking the passenger seat and holding the map.

Our structure is not designed to manage a product, it is designed to manage people, for whom only so much can be controlled or guaranteed. McConnell describes 'quality' as what is built into a product. In the SNF, it can be seen as the 'gift that keeps on giving' (I hate colloquials, but this one really works). Not everybody can see what we see and do what we do and still get up, come back, and do it all over again the next morning.

Further, you'll be challenged to do so when there are differing perspectives to your own, and when decisions are made that you don't necessarily agree with. Hopefully, you'll thrive when under pressure from other powerful members of the team that don't have the same perspectives that you do, or clearly act on a different set of values.

I touched on this briefly when describing the roles of the staff members in Friend or Foe, but here, I'll divulge how a decision is truly made.

Being the newbie, you will not be as confident as you will become later on, but you definitely have potential to take the reins eventually, and people will admire you for doing excellent work. As discussed, this is a process. But entering the SNF with a Capital P mindset will have you failing before you even start.

Why is that?

Power is not static. It grows, it shifts, and in a setting like this, it changes hands often.

Most days are not 'business as usual.' There is a stark difference in the way people do work when it is service-centered rather than production-centered. People come to work for more than just a paycheck, but—ideally—also for more than whatever self-serving reasons they chose the jobs they did.

Although some will complain all the way to pay day and back for numerous years of doing the same job, it is undeniable that many still do the work because there's something about it that makes them feel good.

I believe there is almost always overlap in purpose—another great "p" word—and power. In this overlap, plenty can be lost between the cracks. What may be 'purpose-serving' in essence, could become 'power-serving' on the flip side of the coin. It can look like someone who is apt to take any new or impossible challenge—maybe even those they are not well-equipped to. They do this because it gives them purpose to create solutions and see a better outcome, but also because something about that behavior is exhilarating and the great outcome gives them a right to feel accomplished—to feel powerful.

I don't know that you'll ever be chasing a 'high' like this, but you will have to come to terms with your relationship with power. You'll also have to put your decisions under the microscope before others do. Frequent consideration of this can evade the tug-of-war between power and ethics.

If you guide others one day during their CFY experiences, you have the ability to choose a style of leadership distinct from the way you interact with other staff in the facility that you depend on to see your recommendations and ideas to fruition. You're already a leader when you walk through the glass doorway into the perfidiously quiet, contemporary interior designed lobby of your new, wild experience. But later, you will actually be in charge of someone else's actions. You climb a ladder of sorts, but it's not to be better than anyone. In this case, it's to make someone else better. When you think about your current mentorship, if it's good mentorship, it's possible and very believable that you have someone that works just as hard or harder than you. That's not what we think about when we think of Capital P. In healthcare, we really have to reframe our ideas of power completely to understand who that is and what they look like.

## THE TOP OF THE PYRAMID

While there is a chain of command clear enough to resolve daily issues, our system reflects a balancing act of responsibility and judgement calls. It's less a struggle for power, and more a combined team effort to reach goals. There isn't much room for someone who's concerned about being Capital P. To have humility—the ability to listen, to be corrected, to be wrong—means to be a useful part of the team.

It helps that most people are referred to as "nurse" in this setting, whose job description patients determine to be able to help them with whatever needs they have. As I mentioned in New Guy on the Block (see chapter 5), it's worth it to take on the task to do good things. It reminds you, however, that we are all equals. High school diploma, bachelor's, master's, or doctoral degree. Two years of experience or 30... We all work for the same individuals.

So, guess who Capital P really is. You got that right: "p" is for Patient.

By the way, in the Friend or Foe game (see chapter 6), my rating on patients is always friend. I have made some of the most meaningful friendships I could have dreamed up with someone at least 50 years apart from me by working in a SNF. At what point do the similarities and differences, yelling and laughing, sickness and joy all balance out into just being human with another human, you ask? I say it's all in a therapy session.

When you sit down in a room with a patient, 'position' and 'power' do not translate. In fact, according to an article by Sara Heath, "healthcare professionals are now calling these (paternal) power hierarchies into question, saying that they do not align with patient-centered and value-based healthcare models."[2]

Now, what makes this concept difficult if you're a power seeker? Well, first, not every patient is going to be easily satisfied, nor easy to do good things for. I tend to think that complex medical histories can complicate a person in a way that is not transparent to us. We don't know who they were before, whether they spent more time doing right than wrong, who they voted for, or what their values are. We see someone who is sick, in pain, and in need. So, whoever they were, whoever they are, we are on the other side with flowers and cookies and smiling faces. We try to be who we think they need in a difficult moment, or in the absence of family, to care for them the way they deserve.

"What I say, goes!" is hardly ever a reasonable or effective way to accomplish this.

# STORY TIME WITH LEANDRA
## *P is for Police*

Leandra was a mild case with a wild side. Although she had always had questionable cognitive functioning, she knew exactly who she was. She was aware of her surroundings, could recognize and name every one of her caregivers, and could engage in daily activities without help, as long as it didn't require getting out of a chair.

But she could go from zero to unmeasurable on an anger meter in less than a second.

When it happened, it was a big commotion. If anyone, staff members and fellow residents alike, did anything she didn't like, she'd demand the highest degree of justice for it and spew off a set of ungodly words to get her point across. Me, though, I was exempt from her fury-or so I thought. She liked me. Until she didn't...

When I received orders to see Leandra for dysphagia therapy, I was... speechless, to say the least.

Now, Leandra didn't have to be a tough case, because her deficits were minimal. However, she hated therapy. Worse, to hand her a plate of puree food was just about as criminal as robbing a corner deli. I was to learn this the hard way. During one of our sessions, I asked Leandra to spit out her gum to do a lingual exercise. It appeared she didn't hear me, and so I moved it to the side with the tongue depressor.

"Call the police!" She uttered angrily.

Taken aback, I asked, "Leandra, what are you talking about?"

"NO! What are you doing? Call the damn police!"

With that, we ended the therapy session.

It's not the best example, but I want to bring across that the tendency to apply a heavy hand will inevitably damper our success with some patients. If you're a power seeker, you may be all too easily frustrated when you're unable to get your way in therapy.

Hell, we almost never get our way in therapy. Do your best to evade responding to negative feelings about this—the consequence is never pretty.

## POWER AND PEOPLE

If you're still considering being a power seeker, you also have to consider who you're exerting your power over. Does it help you achieve a goal?

When we interact with departmental staff—those who don't get paid to make decisions, but instead to see them through—are we carefully considering what their knowledge of the patient is? Are we bossy when we direct others, or do we provide education with meekness and mindfulness?

We are not just healthcare. We are long-term care. In a SNF, decisions aren't made in a vacuum. Learn to think beyond yourself constantly, beyond checkpoints A-Z, and certainly beyond who Capital P is.

We'll get into it more in later chapters, (see Chapter 15—We've Come This Far By Faith) but for now, I want you to consider the nature of our approach. McConnell describes the difference in leadership versus forceful pushing. Helping others to understand the advantage rather than carrying out a view of things that are preconceived and deliberate, even if they aren't right for the situation. With decision-making ability, flexibility and understanding sometimes fall into second place. So, the question is, are we trying to get things done through people or trying to get people to do things?[3]

What about those in supervisor or director positions? Where do their intentions lie?

A person who is overly concerned with power will inevitably be corrected by a system that has more power than they can muster. Even though the healthcare system is based on managing people and using cooperative motivation, there is one tangible aspect... the money! You, who have the patient's best interest at heart, will cross paths with those who have the organization's best interest at heart. When that happens, it can present some push back. At a point that you feel pressured, if not entirely shaken into compromise, you should lend primary attention to the quality of your work and ethics. It's a good time to access the Capital P within yourself when you have to fight for what's right .

'Compromise' isn't a bad word, really. However, not all compromises are good. Consider that the goals you have set for your patients are based on what the patient wants and needs in order to fulfill a high quality of life in a setting that is to become their home. These needs are not negotiable. Imagine being in your own home, and being unable to say what you want and when you want it, what you don't want, and when you'd prefer to skip an activity or two. Imagine that those delegated to help you are people who are simply trying to overcome you to keep their own sense of power or their interests satisfied—or worse, to keep someone else whom they answer to satisfied.

If we can't consider ourselves as agents for a greater cause than keeping the wheels turning in our facilities, then maybe we don't differ so much in our industry from corporate environments as we think we do. Don't put people too out of their way and keep calm.

Accept instructions from those 'higher up' and delegate to those 'lower down' on the totem pole.

So, where does power really lie?

This is a personal thing that I want you to write out for yourself. It isn't anything more than you telling yourself who you see in your network—your system.

Who makes the big moves?

_____

_____

When they speak, do you see others back down or give way?

_____

_____

Do you feel like this person is a leader or a commander?

_____

_____

_____

Do you respect their approach?

_____

_____

_____

Do you think it benefits not only your department or your position, but the patient population to whom all of this trickles down?

_____

_____

_____

Do your patients get the last say?

_____

_____

_____

Reflect on your own access to and relationship with 'power' in your workplace.

_____

_____

_____

_____

**CHAPTER FOOTNOTES**

[1]McConnell, Charles. "The Effective Health Care Supervisor 6th Ed. 'Health Care: How Is It Different from 'Industry'?'." Jones & Bartlett Learning, LLC.

http://samples,jbpub.com/9781449604714/04714_CH02_FINAL.pdf.

[2]Heath, Sara. "Understanding the Power Hierarchy in Patient-Provider Relationships." PatientEngagementHIT, July 23, 2018.

https://patientengagementhit.com/news/understanding-the-power-hierarchy-in-patient-provider-relationships.

[3]McConnell, Charles. "The Effective Health Care Supervisor 6th Ed. 'The Nature of Supervision: Health Care & Everywhere'." Jones & Bartlett Learning, LLC.

# 8

# CLOCK IN, WORK, CLOCK OUT

## A Guide to Productivity

Now that you know everybody, it's time to settle in and get comfortable.

You have a job to do, which you'll be expected to get very accustomed to very quickly. I'm sure you've heard about productivity in the medical and rehab arena of the field. It's quite a big deal. I struggled in my first few months to achieve 80% productivity, but in time, I managed about 95% on a good day and actually left when I clocked out. Here's what I found to play a big part in this:

**PREPARE**

The first 15 minutes I spent in the building, I settled in, finding out about any major changes in my patients' care, calculating what documentation I needed to finish by the day's end, and anticipating my patients' diet changes before I put them on paper. I would even fill out orders and organize other paperwork to file at the proper time. After some back and forth at my facility, I made requests for the kitchen at the start of my day. It allowed me the opportunity to avoid wasted time, which kept me focused and my feet moving at a good pace.

A lot of speech-language pathologists have a way of 'scheduling' their day. For instance, in my first 15 minutes, I decided on two people, maybe three, whom I could see for their lunch meals. Otherwise, I just anticipated who I would see in the morning and who I would see in the afternoon. Since my day started at 9 AM, I could easily still have been at work for the supper meal if I had a large caseload.

While you can outline your day, it is very important to remain flexible and make space for things not going the way you expect it to. On an average day, I was turned away 2–3 times due to someone being cleaned up or showering, being in the bathroom, being in another type of rehab therapy, being at an activity (e.g., church), or any other variety of activity that made them unavailable for speech therapy.

It's never worth it to wait for patients to finish their alternative activities. As for using the bathroom, it's not your expected two minutes for 'number one', or 10 minutes max for 'number two'. Assume it will take the entire day, and just go back later. Productivity counts on you! You may also be cut short on your therapy for such reasons; and while it can upset your flow, it's best to split the session or gently ask for five more minutes when reasonable and possible.

The line is fine between a staff member that really needs to handle a certain task at a certain time, and one that is unfair to you and your right to provide therapy. Sometimes, just after sitting down at my patient's side and lifting the spoon to do PO (oral) trials—BAM! A CNA would come strolling in. With nothing more than a three-word sentence grumbled under her breath, she'd whisk my patient away. Inconsiderate as it may be, it happens all the time. It's really best just to allow it at times. There's the whole 'putting yourself in someone else's shoes' thing, and it might be best for the CNA and the patient if they can do bathrooming at that given time or get started on their day. However, you still have the right to insist that the patient complete their therapy session, if this is best for them.

You'll face countless such challenges; therefore, it's important to get creative to offset the least expected turn of events. In a case that you think you have nothing else to do with your time, which is unlikely, consider a few options: see another patient, do some documentation early, do quarterly or annual patient screens, assist or discuss relevant case material with other care providers, take an earlier lunch break, start an earlier lunch with another patient, collect new therapy materials (you know you need to), or with the permission of the rehab director, shorten your therapy time for that day and exercise better communication strategies for the future.

## STORY TIME WITH FEZ
# *My Patients are Busier than Me*

One day, as I entered Fez's room for therapy, he was in the middle of being cleaned by a CNA. By then I knew well that this could easily take another twenty minutes, maybe more. Thus I decided to do a separate session.

Upon my return, I was happy to see him freshly done, waiting in his geri chair. Normally, I would have cringed inwards upon discovering that the CNA still had to brush his teeth... Another two-minute delay! However, this actually worked in my favor. He was on thick-liquids and aspiration precautions because of oropharyngeal dysphagia. Watching his teeth being brushed would give me the perfect opportunity to assess his lingual, mandibular, and labial range of motion, and whether he could tolerate a rinse with thin liquids. I used the time to educate the CNA by suggesting she use a smaller portion of water, or remove most of the toothpaste residue with an oral swab, since this would help avoid the use of more water.

Finally, I could finish my session with Fez. Relieved, I sat down. Of course, when house cleaning barged in and demanded to clean the room, I could do nothing but get up, walk out, and welcome yet another delay with a smile.

## TAKE THE STEPS

Medical speech-language pathology life, I have to be honest, is not for you if you don't enjoy a mildly horrific walk up, down, and back up the same few flights of steps daily. Elevators have been the least functional or productive thing in any medical setting that I know of. What may make them useful are transportation of patients and kitchen items throughout the day. Otherwise, it exists for no apparent or consistent reason, other than being gravely annoying with its persistent faultiness. One day, the elevator at one of my facilities held me hostage for fifteen minutes while I held a patient's hot lunch in my hands. If your facility doesn't have at least a third elevator, you may be better off saving your breath for the steps. I promise you'll accomplish a lot more.

## KNOW YOUR FACILITY'S SCHEDULES

Every Tuesday, we had hairdressing at my primary facility. If I had a patient who enjoyed getting his or her hair done, I didn't even think of planning anything important—like a full meal tray. In fact, if I didn't get to see them first thing in the morning, I just bumped them to the end of my list. On the other hand, if the activity had a set start and finish time, like church, I could plan around it.

Each facility has its floor/wing schedules for meals. If you know that the 6th floor gets their lunch delivered last, you wouldn't show up fifteen minutes too early, just because. Instead, you can easily do an entire meal tray with someone on the 2nd floor, if that floor gets its meals delivered first. If you're unsure, follow up with the kitchen to find out what they've sent up already. I used to pick up my meals directly from the kitchen, but if that is not convenient or allowed at your facility, know that it isn't worth it to wait for meals, even if you know that each day the cart comes up at a certain time. Meals can be late, and it doesn't help to call the kitchen to rush them. Instead, you can work on exercises until the delivery comes or quickly see another patient for a split session. Be aware that meals can also come early. This is part of the reason for informing the nursing staff that you plan to work with a patient at that time, so they don't start without you.

I evaded these issues by having schedules set up with my kitchen. That way, I used the lunch meal time as efficiently as possible.. If I found myself lucky enough to have several patients on one floor, waiting for a meal tray to come up with the cart made sense and worked out better for me and my patients.

## USE SESSION TIME TO EDUCATE

I never realized just how much time you waste on activities which patients aren't good at and won't improve with until I was months into my CFY. I learned that there is instead an opportunity to train the care providers, who will ultimately make the most difference for the patient. Why do passive oral motor exercises for 30 minutes, only to use your non-productive time to communicate if all the patient will respond to, is strategies? You must talk to care providers and nursing staff, anyway; and if the patient is present, you can bill for it. Further, it's necessary that you observe whether they carry the strategies over.

## ACTUALLY WRITE THINGS DOWN

Write down everything! Even if you think you might never look at it again, it will help you to remember it. If it's even remotely important to do, you can see it right next to your schedule and choose a convenient time to attend to it. This can be anything from reporting something non-emergent to another staff member, to updating your PEG tube screens, to printing out documentation.

I developed the habit of writing things down that I had done already, too. This ensured that I followed up with it. An example is when I would put in an order, I usually informed the dietician, the kitchen directors, the nursing supervisors, and the CNAs. That's a lot of people to keep up with, so I made sure I touched all bases.

I even wrote down how my patients responded to each session, just for my personal use. I always found it useful that I could scroll back a couple of days to put a date to significant events for progress notes.

Writing down everything is a valuable practice I still use every day.

Your facility may or may not require that you take daily notes. However, I encourage you to do it, anyway.

## STAY PACKIN'

As you can expect, you'll spend much of the day around food. Carrying a lunch box or having really big pockets is helpful for carrying snacks and miscellaneous tools around the building, helping you avoid several trips or calls to the kitchen. Do be aware of where and how to store food, as you don't want to be out of compliance with the Department of Health (DOH) standards. Cover your drinks when walking with them in the halls and always have perishable items refrigerated in the pantry. Do not leave anything unsealed unattended.

## DON'T EXTEND SESSION TIME

It may be tempting to continue on when you're having a great outcome during a session. Perhaps it took an entire 25 minutes for your patient to cooperate. We're not the only profession that relies on being extremely timely. If you're seeing a mental health therapist, you might be at the climax of your heartbreaking story. The therapist will tell you to stop immediately and continue the next time. It sucks, but it's a part of what the job requires of us. I struggle most when I see patients for lunch. If I know the patient eats slowly enough to take more than 30 minutes to finish, I make sure I bring a lunch of their current consistency and change it out with the more advanced consistency before leaving him or her to continue. You could also plan to have more than one patient in the same dining room so you can see both within the combined, designated contact time.

## TAKE YOUR BREAKS WISELY

With a full caseload, it becomes quite difficult to avoid sluggishness in the workplace. We aren't exactly working with kids who will keep us on our feet, nor do we have a live clown show (unless the activities department tries to outdo themselves). Drink your water and eat some of those cookies you'd otherwise be offering to your patients.

I used to pair my lunch with paperwork and an imaginary glass of wine. It saved so much time on documentation. You may consider your lunchtime to be more sacred than I. I don't recommend you lose out on that time to scroll on Instagram or whatever is relaxing for you in that 30-minute period, if you don't want to. Whatever works for you, works.

## STAY ON TOP OF YOUR DOCUMENTATION

Speaking of the devil, it can get out of hand very quickly if you wake up to eight progress notes due on the same day. You always have the option to do some of it earlier than the due date, and might prefer it to being extremely late. I'll note that progress notes and evaluations typically have a 24 or 48 hour grace period, but orders, chart notes, and recertifications do not. Technically, you are not paid to do documentation, and you do not want to be stuck at work off the clock, trying to finish it all up at once.

## OUTLINE YOUR PAPERWORK

Repetitiveness is a synonym to the field of SLP. Your patients are not so different that you can't have a general sense of phrasing for your referral justifications and pick-ups, your goals, and your care planning. Take the time to be more specific where and when necessary to ensure that someone else reading it is well-enough informed, and that one patient's case doesn't look exactly like another's.

## LEARN YOUR SHORT-HAND

If you work at a paper-based facility, you may feel like you're in over your head when trying to decipher scribbles and short-hand abbreviations. Some have more than one meaning and sometimes spelling errors happen, so it is important to overcome obfuscation and ambiguity by considering the context and asking questions when you need clarification.

It's not my style to use too much short-hand when using a digital EMR. For well-recognized diagnoses, such as SOB or HTN, I don't mind. I'll use it for thickened liquid consistencies, as well. Otherwise, I find it easier to spell things out when I'm typing.

## 'BUILD' YOUR NOTES

Your digital EMR may offer ways for you to 'build' a section of your notes by clicking through a successive pattern with multiple lists of sentence fragments for each section to outline precautions, make an order, or state a goal.

Again, I fall on the opposite end of this one. If I don't have to build a note, I most often won't. I've outlined and memorized my statements so well, I custom create them as a habit. When I use the build function, it also reduces my motivation to be specific in places I should.

You may consider some of these options to make your day go by just a bit quicker. What quirks have you found that help you get through the day productively?

_____

_____

_____

_____

Productivity is the single most important thing your facility cares about when it comes to rehab therapy. This advice is to help you do a great job with all the skills you've learned in school, while looking like you have it all together and managing an expectation that can seem through the roof at first.

# Part Three
## SNF PROCEDURES AND PROCESSES

# 9

# TIDBITS

## A Guide to the Swallow Evaluation

The swallow evaluation is among the many things you will master during your CFY. You will never be a gold standard MBS, but you will notice that your visualization of the swallow process and your inclinations get better and better every day. I won't brag, but I can now analyze a swallow to an extent that surprises me, even on the phone with a friend who is eating or drinking.

## FIRST, THE CHART REVIEW

You will become familiar with some patients you evaluate and have the general rundown of their diets, medical histories, and what they're allergic to. Clearly, you will never know what changes they may present with when you go to see them, especially if the person consulting you shows a decline in function. When dealing with a patient you've never met, you need all points touched on, even the stuff that seems irrelevant. Seeing a patient before reading a chart poses no true use to your evaluation and can have undesirable outcomes if you miss something important. Note that there are some differences between a post-acute speech or swallow evaluation and an in-house evaluation, and it's mostly the subjective portions.

### Post-Acute

In the patient review instrument (PRI), the document that comes with the patient from their acute setting, I looked primarily for:

- Admitting diagnosis and prior medical history.
- Discharge diet.
- Previous bedside swallow evaluation.
- Previous objective swallow evaluation.
- Radiology imaging.

- Surgeries.
- Allergies.

Some also look at blood and urine labs for albumin, BUN, RBC and WBC count. Secondary to the patient's medical status, but necessary for the write-up, would be the patient's age, living situation, and length of hospital stay.

## In-House

To see a patient who is a long-term resident or a resident not picked up for therapy days after admission and initial screening, I looked for:

- Nursing notes regarding the reason for consultation (3 consecutive days, if a non-emergent case, such as a possible diet upgrade).
- Verbal communication with the nursing staff and supervisor.
- PRI for any recent hospitalization.
- New diagnoses or new medications.
- Previous speech/swallow therapy documentation.
- Current diet and supplements.
- Alertness.
- Weight gain or loss.

There is certainly some overlap here, as a long-term patient can be hospitalized and sent back to the facility on a completely different diet. Ideally, you would treat this patient as a new admission and check all points, since realistically, you would not know what has changed. You want to see these patients as soon as you can because when someone returns to the facility, and everyone is familiar with them, it sometimes goes back to business as usual. So, you want to offer your recommendation or training before the day really starts, to avoid mistakes on the part of the caregivers or nursing staff who are familiar with the patient.

## Gather your materials:

- Tongue depressor.
- Lemon glycerin swabs.
- Pipettes.
- Paper towels.
- Extra cup.
- Spoons.
- Gloves.
- Applesauce.
- Soft Cookie, Graham Cracker, or bread.
- Saltine Cracker.

- Optional: Straw.
- Optional: Stethoscope.

For food trials, the food mentioned in the list can be replaced with anything of the same consistency. If you aren't sure, the dietician is a good person to ask about the division of consistencies on kitchen items.

## THE ASSESSMENT

It may be best to trial liquids first, followed by solids. There is always a possibility that with solid trials, the patient may need liquids to assist with softening the food or washing the mouth of residue after swallowing. Trial only the consistencies you assume the patient would be able to consume without choking. For instance, if there is a lot of coughing with a more restrictive consistency, you shouldn't advance. If nectar-thick liquids are difficult, water would presumably be much more difficult. Keep in mind that water is unlike other thin liquids in the sense that it has no taste or stimulation. Some people with oropharyngeal deficits will respond differently to juice than to water for this reason. There is no true need to trial both, but if you assume the person is more at risk, clear water is better to get a baseline measure while avoiding complication of aspiration. One may also take the precaution of doing a thicker liquid trial first or instilling precautionary measures (e.g., the use of a teaspoon as opposed to a cup or straw).

Your purpose during the swallow evaluation is to assess each level of the patient's swallow and determine which levels present with dysfunction. As you provide trials, the best thing you can do is to use digital palpation. I included a stethoscope in the materials list so as to suggest that you may have been trained to do cervical auscultation. If so, and it is something you feel comfortable with, simply outline in your documentation that you used this and the details of the results this method of testing provided you. Keep in mind that cervical auscultation alone does not allow you to assess oral levels of the swallow and may not be transparent to all pharyngeal functions either, such as hyolaryngeal elevation. Better than traditional methods, cervical auscultation may allow you to assess breathing patterns in alternation with the swallow.

After all is said and done, ensure your patient's mouth is completely clear. There is nothing worse you can do than leave a patient—especially one that is not alert—with oral debris that places them at a risk of aspirating after you have left the room. Always note oral clearance in your documentation and describe how it was achieved. There is really no reason to forget or miss this step.

## DOCUMENTATION

What I share on documentation in this section will apply to any evaluation write-up, with just a few variations. I've already gone through how to write for you and your patients, but how does that really look when writing a swallow evaluation?

Go into the documentation only after fully considering everything you've witnessed during your sit-down with the patient. You will have to create a diagnosis for the patient and then justify it. This can get a bit tricky if you're used to placing a diagnosis at the end, when discussing your clinical impressions on paper. I am careful to choose my diagnosis first when using an EMR, because otherwise I get jumbled up in the percentages and skill levels that are pre-populated in the system, leading me to specify a severity level or type of dysphagia that's not necessarily a good depiction of my patient.

I'll explain a bit more.

You may have a patient with whom you trialed puree. When you presented the puree, the patient had bolus holding and, when you gave them some cueing and stimulation, they swallowed it. You noticed about one or two seconds that the patient had an effortful initiation to swallow the bolus. The swallow was also noticeably loud. There were no hyolaryngeal elevation problems and no coughing. You looked in the patient's mouth and saw a part of the bolus still there. The patient had swallowed 90% of the bolus, which was small to begin with, so he didn't have severe oral clearance problems, but after giving him sips of water, he still couldn't completely clear it, so you had to whip out your handy dandy pipette and clean the patient's mouth.

Here's one problem with documenting that: at least on the EMR that I use, 1 to 2 seconds delayed is within functional limits (WFL). Do you know how long 1 to 2 seconds feels when you're trying to swallow something? That is not functional at all! It can take less than two seconds to aspirate before effectively triggering a swallow, but according to your EMR, this person has no pharyngeal deficits. Further, there is no pre-populated selection for an audible swallow, which is not itself a deficit but can indicate something that is, such as a delay.

The next problem with documenting this observation is when the patient doesn't present the same way with each swallow of the same consistency. The oral clearance was fair but was non-functional beyond the initial swallow. My EMR will prompt me to indicate whether I see this as mild, moderate, or severe. It really depends. I will have to decide based on my overall observation, including additional trials. Perhaps I'll have to average out the ones that were functional and those that were notably impaired. I would likely also note whether the dysfunction observed after an initially okay swallow was suspected to be related to fatigue, a need for additional stimulation, absent dry swallow, etc.

To not tangent too much, when you're writing up your evaluation documentation, stay a step ahead and be a little smarter than your EMR. You will certainly have to fill in gaps.

I know this because I move around sometimes: some SLPs are 100% trained to the EMR, and if it doesn't blink and beep red when you attempt to save it, it's completed.

NO, sis.

I have a strong pet peeve, and it's when SLPs document like they weren't even in the room when this evaluation happened.

My pointers are:

## TAKE ADVANTAGE OF EVERY LITTLE BOX

This doesn't apply when your EMR asks you for your patient's hobbies during your write-up of a dysphagia evaluation. If Tom's favorite activity isn't hot dog eating contests, I frankly don't think it has any place on the evaluation. I surely don't have 'hobbies' on the list of things I'm asking my patient about when I enter the room with a dysphagia consult, so feel free to skip those kinds of boxes. Don't skip those that ask about your patient's previous tests, X-rays, and encounters with other health and medical professionals, especially GI or ENT. If the patient's PRI contains an MBS, get a binder or folder and treasure it; you won't see many of those that you don't ask for, and even then...

## TAKE THE EVALUATION SERIOUSLY

Face it: we SLPs may think we know it all, and we can already envision what's going to happen when we walk into a room. We are tempted to trial two consistencies, when really, we should have trialed three. Maybe we skip over applying a few strategies or maneuvers during the evaluation. With documentation, it's important that if you say something happened or is likely to happen, there is something behind that. Don't cut corners, because you will spend the next 4 weeks of therapy making up for horrible goals and crappy baselines.

## DON'T LIMIT YOURSELF

Keep in mind that your evaluation reflects your view of and actual plan for this patient. Despite placing orders for four weeks of therapy, your therapy may only really need to last a week. Am I going to write 16 goals for someone that I will see for one week? No. Am I going to write goals that won't reasonably be reached in that one week? No. My point is not to limit yourself, but to have you be more abreast of your plan, so that your action follows through with that.

## DOCUMENT EVERYTHING, EVEN IF IT SEEMS INSIGNIFICANT

While you don't have to, I recommend documenting even minor cognitive deficits or speech- and voice-related problems you notice during the dysphagia evaluation, and justify why you would not pick up at the defined time. I also outline that I will continue to follow up with the patient and nursing staff on the issue. This lends itself to the plan—to follow up later—and also to the total view of the patient.

## **GOAL WRITING**

Here's the fun part... From what you've learned during the assessment, what are the most useful things you can anticipate the patient improving on and through what medium or at what level of assistance?

Well first, what did you notice? Does your patient have an oral phase or a pharyngeal phase dysphagia, or both? In which phase are the deficits more prominent? This may determine how to divide your time during the course of therapy. Thirty minutes can feel like a lifetime, or it can go by in a finger snap. Dysphagia therapy tends to be the former for me, but at times, when I would see some progressive accomplishment with a patient—boom—I would glance at the clock only to see that 30 or more minutes had passed.

Whenever I chose my goals in the SNF, I thought of the patient's level of independence, ability to follow directions, self-awareness and ability to self-correct during the task, consistency, and their expected ability to carry-over new strategies. Now, this part isn't really teachable. You will get to know what types of boxes you can check for the patients you see; much of it is common sense, though.

To write a goal, you must consider what your patient presents like and what you need them to accomplish to move closer to a normal level of functioning. If you think your patient won't achieve a super-high level of functioning, don't place that into your goal (even the long-term goal).

Now, you can write. If you use an EMR that allows you to build your goal, you may prefer to let it guide you. Disclaimer: This synopsis is from my experience of using Rehab Optima. With the use of another EMR, the steps may differ, just as the level and quality of guidance on the system can also differ. However, your goal should look about the same at the end.

The platform may first give you the option to 'build' your goal based on areas of your assessment you marked below a functional level. Maybe you marked mastication as mild, moderate, or severe. The EMR may give you a goal that says, "Patient will improve mastication to _____(level of achievement), with _____(level of assistance or cueing), to improve ability to _____ (long-term goal or patient's ideal situation)."

The benefit of using the 'build' option is that when the patient has achieved the goal, you can upgrade the goal easily by changing your achievement level and level of assistance. Your justification or reason for aiming towards this particular goal typically will not change in this situation.

If it ever is so that your justification changes, you should state it very clearly within the documentation, not just the goal writing.

If you're like me, you prefer to write out your goals from scratch because... well, something about homemade pie just tastes sweeter than Entenmanns. I don't really like pre-packaged pie, just like I don't like pre-packaged goals. I won't lie, though, I've stolen some wording or even therapy ideas from the 'build' section—with a SNF population, you sometimes feel run dry and like you don't even know what you know. Anyway, when I'm writing my goals, I find it quick and easy to just write exactly what I want to write.

Let's start with the long-term goal, as you will base short-term goals on that.

I would typically split it up between a liquid consistency and a solid consistency. Some may write a general 'least restrictive diet' goal; that's fine too. Sometimes, the patient's fundamental problem is that they don't eat enough. If that's the case, your goal will outline 'optimal PO intake.'

Short-term goals will refer to the long-term goals indirectly. Generally, to manage the least restrictive diet, you want to improve all areas of the swallow that are impacted by the dysphagia problem: mastication, hyolaryngeal elevation, and oral clearance. Outline the specific exercises and techniques you hope to use to obtain achievement towards the long-term goal. When you see an improvement in the therapeutic activities, you at least hope it makes a difference in how the patient tolerates oral trials and meals.

Remember: your silent goal is to reduce both the patient's and caregiver's burden, therefore it's important to consider who cares for this patient and what they are capable of.

Depending on who signs your paperwork, you'll have to write goals their way. Just when you thought grad school was over! I won't do you the injustice of writing goals for you, for two reasons. One, I am not your clinical supervisor and I don't seek to provide you with the guidance they are meant to. I only want to give you tips and a greater understanding of what to expect, based on what I've experienced. I don't want angry letters from you telling me how I've made you piss off said supervisor because you did it alternatively to her teaching. Second, I truly don't think there's a right way and that every other way is wrong, like many of your graduate clinical supervisors and clinical writing goblins may have made you believe. As long as what's expected is understood, you've done just fine. You can take the reins from there.

## ORDERS & CARE PLAN

Orders, orders, orders.

They are arguably the most important, yet simplest part of this process. Your orders will outline what you intend to do during the therapy course and how much time you need. The orders are not flexible like the goals are: these remain the same for the entire therapy course. Note that if you recertify and have new goals for speech and language, not just dysphagia—you will need additional orders for that. In some facilities, you will even need to renew your four-week order, as it's not automatic, so just check in.

How I've learned to write my orders for dysphagia therapy:

*ST Tx for dysphagia 3-5x weekly for 4 weeks to facilitate improved swallow function for least restrictive diet.*

I would change this wording ever so infrequently; in special cases, where 'least restrictive diet' was not definitive enough, or the patient's physical swallow function was actually not the source of their problem, I would write "improve oral intake" or "for return to/tolerance of previous level of functioning (PLOF) consistency, as appropriate."

You will most likely be the responsible party in placing the order for diet consistency (if not the dietitian, nursing supervisor, or physician—it depends on the facility). It will be important to keep all diet restrictions the same that are unrelated to your scope. For example, your patient may have a list of allergies, a fluid restriction, and a low-fat diet; you will only make changes to the diet consistency (e.g., upgrade to chopped solids and thin liquids). You may include allowances for specific items from an advanced diet consistency, as well.

Care planning is the next step, and just as simple. Somewhere in the patient's chart, there is a specific form for this. Perhaps it's electronic at your facility. Basically, it outlines when you've begun a therapy plan for your patient and why. When the therapy course ends, you sign and date that too. Sometimes—but rarely—you might find yourself outlining in the care plan. The changes you make are on a case-by-case, facility-by-facility basis. It could reflect a diet upgrade, a decrease in function, or the specification of a strategy or precaution that needs to be consistently applied for the patient's care to be followed through appropriately.

The funny little thing about a therapeutic care plan for speech is that no one who is expected to carry it out, i.e., the nursing staff, really read it. Your true care plan is word of mouth. Communicating with the CNAs is the only way to apply the necessary techniques you wish to use to facilitate improved function for your patient. So besides checking all of your boxes and dotting all of your i's, remember also to smile and make friends; you'll thank them later.

# A Guide to PEG Tube Recommendation and Weaning

When a patient has a gastronomy tube, we proceed with dysphagia therapy in a method distinct from our usual admission or in-house pick ups. These patients' cases are significantly more sensitive because there is a far greater risk of airway protection difficulty, if the gastronomy status is related to dysphagia. Remember that not all PEG tubes are placed for an airway protection problem, and you will need to proceed with caution as to not overlook other risks that may present with oral feeding. A pick up of this sort should be something the physician becomes aware of as soon as you consider it.

## THE CHART REVIEW

When considering an in-house pick up, even if a patient's chart has prior instrumental testing, it really cannot be taken at face value, so I rarely scrounged for details from it, except to document it. If the most recent test was one year ago and showed that the patient could tolerate thin liquids with a head turn, and the patient was discharged from therapy with no pleasure allowances for that, I would take it with a huge grain of salt. The most recent dysphagia evaluation, screening, or therapy document will be more helpful to clarify your justification and therapeutic approach.

While the chart review is the first thing you want to complete in this type of case, don't overlook a conversation with the family. You will benefit from a thorough explanation of the individual's prior functioning to establish your approach to the therapy. This is especially important if you want to reintroduce foods on a pleasure-based schedule, as opposed to simply considering consistency. You want to keep the patient's motivation high, which can be difficult when he or she develops an aversion to food they find hard to eat and relies on the alternative method to keep themselves alive.

The approach to therapy begins with identifying your patient, their history, and the terms of their gastronomy status.

## NEW ADMISSION ON PEG

In the patient review instrument (PRI), I checked in especially for:

- Admitting diagnosis and prior medical history.
- Neurological status.
- Chest X-ray or CT identifying lung status and/or history of aspiration pneumonia.
- Date of PEG placement.
- Diet prior to PEG status.
- Bedside swallow evaluation/treatment notes.
- Instrumental swallow evaluation.
- Alertness.

## 1+ YEARS PEG STATUS

To see a long-term resident or a resident whose admission was not primarily related to PEG status, I looked for similar information to my normal dysphagia evaluation, and checked in especially for:

- Nursing notes regarding reason for consultation.
- Previous speech/swallow therapy documentation.
- Any pleasure feeding.
- Recent weight management.
- Tolerance of PEG tube (reported by CNAs and nurse).
- Alertness.

## THE ASSESSMENT

How long a person has been tube fed will play a major part in your approach to the treatment. It can also yield some assumptions about a prognosis and rehab potential. A new PEG tube is usually placed to manage severe weight loss or to support a patient for an extended time during their recovery after a traumatic event. If swallow therapy is unsuccessful during that time, the PEG status will be extended for years or for the remainder of the patient's lifespan.

A patient with a PEG tube can experience fluctuations in swallow function or may have rehab potential after several years of having no food by mouth. No patient should be written off simply because they have had this means of nutrition for as long as anyone can remember. As discussed in Let's Get Literate, coverage for these feedings will have to be justified yearly. In some facilities, six-month or quarterly screenings will be mandated to ensure that these people do not fall off the radar.

You do want to ensure that the patient is stable, considering their medical diagnoses and weight management. When you start with trials of PO, it might (although not likely) alter their tolerance of the PEG tube feeding or negatively affect their weight. If they seem to struggle with weight continuously, stay in close communication with the multidisciplinary team, including the dietician and physician, to ensure it is the right time to begin your intervention.

The weaning process can be complicated, and the steps you take largely depend on the patient, the family, and the facility. It may seem strange, but agencies and facilities do have rules in place to protect these patients during the process. As a clinical fellow, I was unable to provide PO feeding at the beginning of the PEG tube weaning process. They ridiculed me for it when I spoke to colleagues and during interviews for other jobs. An instrumental assessment, such as an MBS, was required prior to providing any PO. The problem with this was that prior to getting an objective assessment, the patient had to be seen for an average of 2–3 weeks, and I would have to refer him almost immediately upon evaluation with barely any justification. Presenting anything but food (e.g., ice chips or saliva) is less indicative of the true dysphagia problem than actual food, even if it is of a restrictive consistency. The order of things really should be based on your clinical judgement, with the help of your clinical supervisor, to ensure you check all your bases and ensure you're in compliance.

That being said, you would not present PO to a patient that has a PEG tube until you can see some level of ability to swallow it. If your patient does not trigger a swallow, is very lethargic, and barely exhibits a desire for anything like this, it is likely too early to force a spoonful into his or her mouth. This is likely a fragile patient, and each step towards their recovery should be taken with care.

## GOAL WRITING

As you know, PEG tube weaning involves improvement of the patient's swallow function. Therefore, the ideals of the therapeutic process are similar to those outlined in the previous section. There are a few distinctions, though.

For someone with NPO status on a PEG tube, who will not receive any oral nutrition due to a severe dysfunction of their swallow mechanism, your therapy goals can reflect the use of low-risk tasks, such as coating a teaspoon in applesauce or feeding the patient ice chips. This takes into consideration that if any aspiration were to occur, it would not be considerably dangerous. When even low-risk tasks prove difficult or unsafe for the patient during the evaluation, you can center therapy goals around salivary management and then aim for more advanced goals as the patient shows improvement.

The long-term goal will less likely reflect an expectation of achieving a 'least restrictive diet.' For that reason I preferred to use "return to PO intake" as a goal instead, because at the start of this intervention, the most important thing is that the patient will not require the use of the PEG as the sole source of nutrition.

If your patient can tolerate some consistencies upon evaluation, it would certainly help to place a long-term goal towards consuming an entire meal or pleasure feeding of these consistencies. You may choose to outline that the patient will tolerate one meal daily. You may even specify which meal; typically, it would be lunch, or breakfast and lunch when two meals are on the patient's orders. Your clinical judgement, as well as the facility's (specifically the dietary department) procedures, will determine how you organize this in your plan and orders.

## WEANING PLAN

When oral feeding begins (after NPO status), it must be very conservative, meaning small amounts with nicely spaced intervals to assess the swallow completely and note any delayed effects. You may be enthusiastic to trial too much, too quickly, but this can be detrimental. It's best to trial one consistency per session, until adequate intake for an entire meal has been made possible.

It's no rule, but I hate to rely on too many compensatory strategies, maneuvers, and positions to 'make' the feeding work well. Ideally, your patient will show increased strength and coordination to manage at least one soft or smooth consistency that you can stick to for a while to retrain them to accept food in this way. (I use the word "ideally," because there's too many variations and possibilities with each patient, and attention to detail will ultimately help you put one foot in front of the other.) My most successful PEG tube weans happened when the patients felt good. It's not to say that a strategy such as a head turn or chin tuck is a drawback. It's just that sometimes, applying the compensatory strategy is more difficult and less pleasurable for the patient than doing things their way. In the weaning plan, you should look forward to having the patient consume as much as possible, with as much ease as possible.

A patient's family used to cook Dominican food and puree it, as we had decided that was the best consistency for her. This patient had the best outcome with this strategy, considering that the food we served at the facility was not her favorite and she often refused it. It took personalized methods to increase her interest in eating, and even then, keeping her motivated was hard. Your patient's chances of success may increase if their ethnic background can be considered from the start of your therapy intervention—especially if refusal of food is a part of the reason they are on the PEG.

A PEG tube weaning program has the ideal of completely alleviating the need for using the tube, but in this setting you will more often achieve a hybrid (tube and oral) feeding style that the nursing staff, dietician, and speech-language pathologist will manage. For some patients, significant progress will be evident in one course of therapy. For others, progressive changes and additions to an oral diet over several courses of therapy are the best solutions. An overzealous approach may not be in the best interest of every patient, and if a secondary source of feeding is available and safe, you will actually have an advantage throughout the therapeutic process.

## ORDERS & CARE PLAN

Your orders will definitely be for dysphagia therapy when considering a PEG tube weaning program. However, your facility may specify a modality specific to this sort of treatment. It might be a stretch, and I can't say that I've done this, but if your treatment includes a significant amount of training to understand this new situation and adjust the patient to caring for the PEG tube and feeding appropriately, whether that be remembering the right times and the sequential process (especially if they'll be discharged with it after short-term care), this can be considered a cognitive approach, of sorts. Most often, however, the patient will not be responsible for this because the nursing staff will manage it entirely. Even if the patient goes home with it, the process typically changes from a pump method (by machine) to a bolus feeding method, which requires the person to use gravity or a syringe to pass the formula through the tube. The family receives extensive training prior to the patient's discharge, as the patient is typically not independent in this task and may be bound to a chair or bed. As I always say, each situation is unique and decisions will be made based on what is appropriate for the patient, so take it all with a grain of salt.

In your diet orders, you always want to ensure that you recommend the continued use of PEG tube feeding, whether as a primary or supplemental source of nutrition and hydration. You must be very clear in your documentation and orders when you no longer feel the patient benefits from continued use of this. Also, this will only occur after discussions with the dietitian and physician.

While this section is dedicated to discussing the process of creating a therapeutic plan for weaning a patient away from the PEG tube, be mindful that your initial swallow evaluation may indicate severe deficits that can make any oral diet unsafe for the patient. The decision to place a PEG tube is never the responsibility of a single professional and, of course, requires the family's consent. It is certainly a team effort. However, the patient who does not have a tube placed as yet may become a candidate for one (this requires the speech-language pathologist's documentation of the evaluation and justification). Your referral process for this will obviously follow, starting with the nursing supervisor. If immediate discharge to the hospital is not an option, it will be necessary to identify how this patient will be sustained after you leave the room; this will be outlined in the orders, as well. If some other method (e.g., IV fluid) cannot sustain your patient while therapy and observation ensue, orders for the most restrictive diet are expected.

When it comes to PEG tube care and management, communication is all the more important. Your patient does not benefit from any part of the care team 'not knowing' what's going on. That is a sure formula for problems to come. Your care plan will experience many changes along the way, even more complex than for typical dysphagia treatment. It is more important to document what is going on, who you have conferred with, and what the patient is eating—when, how, and with whom, at what level of assistance and supervision. As many ways as you find to document these, do it.

# A Guide to the Speech-Language Evaluation

If your situation is anything like mine was, you'll frequent the speech-language evaluation and therapy process far less than the swallow evaluation and therapy process. It's something I feel I've not gotten to master nearly as well, but I can share what I've learned, at least.

My approach to speech-language and cognitive-communication therapy differed depending on whether my patients were there for post-acute care, or in-house (long-term) residents.

## FIRST, THE CHART REVIEW

The chart review is important—no matter what the situation is. In fact, while they're on therapy, make a habit of sporadic reviews of your patients' charts. I'll get back to this in Do I Have to Call? (chapter 10), but for now, I'll focus on what you should look for in the chart for a newly consulted patient.

### Post-Acute

- Primary diagnosis and prior medical history, specifically for dementia, stroke, Parkinson's Disease, Respiratory issues, Cardiac Issues, Developmental Disorders, and Intellectual Disorders.
- Prior level of functioning (should, but is not always available in the PRI).
- Orientation (to be compared with current functioning).
- Medications.
- Family information.
- Brief Interview of Mental Status (BIMS) score (administered, usually by the social worker, upon admission).
- Presence of other ST-related deficits (like dysphagia).

## In-house

- Nursing notes of a change in function, whether it's an increase or decrease.
- Alertness of the patient and his/her stimulability.
- Medication changes.
- New diagnoses.
- Non-English native language (we won't lie to ourselves here, language therapy is going to be a hell of a difficult thing to provide if we aren't bilingual).
- Previous therapy and success rate.
- Success in other therapies.
- Family involvement.
- Patient awareness of and interest in his/her deficits.
- Insurance and necessity for other therapy (Med B).
- Dependence on ventilator/trach.
- Sensory abilities (like blindness).
- Presence of other ST-related deficits (like dysphagia).
- Participation in activities of daily living (ADLs) and social activities.

I want to point out how long that list was. It may help you understand why it's more difficult to justify speech-language or even cognitive-communication therapy in a long-term setting.

If a patient's change in function is clearly because of a medication change, the solution is not speech therapy. Likely, the new medication makes the patient non-alert, even lethargic, and that is beyond what you should feel you have to overcome. Until the patient is fit for rehabilitative measures, the clinician may decide to defer treatment (or even evaluation) in a case such as this.

Obviously, if your patient doesn't speak the language you speak—or it's not their first—it will further complicate the case, as you need to figure out what the actual needs of the patient are. Perhaps they don't have a receptive language problem, they just don't understand the nursing staff's dialect. Perhaps they don't have a word-finding problem, they just don't know that word in English. The family can be a great help, but also having an interpretation system of some sort, like using the staff around you for assistance, is key to gain a better understanding of the patient's situation. You'll most likely have to figure out a more concrete and reliable system on your own, especially if your facility doesn't offer an interpretation system.

When considering the patient's previous therapies (including other rehab therapies), think about how much you can expect the patient to achieve. The patient's interest and success in those therapies usually carry over in this case. The past is not just the past. This does not necessarily apply to swallow therapy, but it applies to speech.

Sensory disabilities change the way you can cue the patient. As an example, visual cues won't work for a blind person. Though we are used to providing visual cues and materials to stimulate the patient for speech, we have to consider how else we will get through our therapy.

Insurance is a general consideration, especially if the patient requires any testing beyond your scope. If the patient or his or her family pays privately for their stay and access to services, you will need to know if they care to have and pay for your service, and for how long. Your rehab director will also consider the division of treatment among rehab services. For instance, if the patient needs more physical therapy, but their whole allowance has gone into speech therapy, the director will have to pull some strings to make that feasible for the patient. I'll talk about this more in PDPM. Depending on the insurance, the patient may also be eligible to receive additional time for sessions if they need extra attention. Insurance may also determine whether the patient can be seen as a part of a speech group rather than through individual sessions only.

When the patient has additional deficits that are ST-related, the weighing out of the therapy time is crucial. Keep in mind that 30 minutes is not a lot of time. If the patient's primary motive is to wean from a PEG tube, working for even half of that time on speech inevitably reduces the efficiency with which you will reach towards the primary motive. For post-acute patients, I would typically pick up for dysphagia first, and then speech-language and cognitive-communication afterwards, depending on the severity and source of the speech problem. The reason for this is that the speech—or, more often, cognitive—problem may be related to the medical diagnosis or medication, and patients are still recovering when they arrive at the facility. A stroke is not the only diagnosis with a spontaneous recovery of speech and communication abilities. As long as you are seeing the patient, you may do continuous screening and informal activities, and if increasing alertness does not resolve the problem, you may recertify the patient with additional goals.

## GATHER YOUR MATERIALS

- Blank paper.
- Pen.
- Speech-language assessment form.
- Cognitive-communication assessment form.
- Objective batteries as appropriate and timely.
- Picture flash cards.
- ADL items.
- Scene picture.
- Pre-written short story (with questions).

## THE ASSESSMENT

Consider that if the patient wears hearing aids, these must be tested for functionality before you begin with the evaluation. A way to screen hearing aid efficiency informally—as there is no machine nor audiologist on site—is to phonate single high and low frequency speech sounds behind a thin screen which will avoid distorting the sound and not allow your patient to see your mouth.

The speech evaluation takes a significantly longer time to complete than the swallow evaluation, so notify your director if you need him to allot more time for you to do that, especially if you are doing a dysphagia evaluation, as well. You don't want to spend two hours doing any evaluation, really, but it's best not to have too much therapy on top of that, which would make it difficult to manage your day.

It helps to prepare the patient for what to expect when starting the evaluation. It will reduce the chances of responses like, "Why are you asking me these things?" You may stick to the assessment form to a tee; or add, change, or subtract as you need to. It is informal and will not affect the overall view of the patient. However, you should be careful to include each section and create similar and culturally appropriate examples.

Your purpose is not to overwhelm the patient. If they have a lot of trouble completing a simple task, there is no reason to give them a more complex one. If they aren't able to answer a question, and you've already given them a few cues, notate and move on. If the patient is or becomes significantly tired during the evaluation, complete it later in the day, if possible. The answer is to use your judgement and worry most about finding a baseline and potential to make improvement with your assistance.

While you will give some cues during the evaluation, there's no need to do too much just to have the patient succeed, because the therapy time is dedicated to helping the patient achieve success. The evaluation creates a baseline and helps you learn what kinds of cues are useful for the patient. If they don't mimic models or even make eye contact, you will naturally consider using a different level or type of assistance, which you will state in your goal.

It's also helpful to ask questions that are not a direct part of the assessment as you go along. These can include a question such as, "Have you ever seen this before?" If the patient has never seen a windmill, they won't know what to call it. You don't want to deduce that a patient has a word-finding problem when the culprit is really the lack of exposure to an item. Specific, well-formulated questions can help you avoid miscalculating a patient's abilities in the way of descriptions or literacy. Examples are: "Can you see this entire picture?" or, "Is this print big enough for you?"

A patient may ask, "Am I doing okay?" Did I do that right?" I preferred not to respond to too many of these questions when I did evaluations. It's not a rule, and sometimes I gave the patient the correct response after they gave an incorrect one. What's most useful for your time is to wait until the assessment is complete so that you can give the patient a general run-down of what you noticed and general goals you will look towards working on. For example, it is adequate to say, "We are going to work on improving your memory and attention."

## GOAL WRITING

From what you've learned during the assessment, what are the most useful things you can anticipate the patient improving in and through what medium or at what level of assistance?

Sound familiar? You got that right.

Speech goals are a far cry from dysphagia goals only in that your long-term goal will reflect an entirely different skill or means of improving the patient's quality of life. Still, you are only following the process of breaking down what you know about the patient, what you know about development or rehabilitation of the skills, and making a baby out of it.

So, what did you notice this time? Given that you've used a comprehensive assessment tool (i.e., it covers a range of skills, including motor speech, expressive language, receptive language, and various areas of cognition), you'll have a great pick of the litter for your therapy goals. Typically, my speech goals were twice the number of my dysphagia goals. While it may seem like an overbearing task to work session-to-session on six goals rather than three, remember two things. One, you don't have to work on each goal every single day. Given that you have five days to treat, you can literally work on one each day of the week, with a cherry on top on Friday.

Ideally, heeding my second point, you can work on multiple goals at once. In my experience, this is not the best approach in dysphagia therapy. I preferred to do everything disjointly when I treated these types of cases: oral on one day, pharyngeal on another day, solids on one day, liquids on another day, and so on. With speech and communication, it's natural for me to take random opportunities as teaching moments for any skill. Working memory and executive function come into play during the use of compensatory strategies for orientation. Yes, by picking up a calendar and finding the right date, you're already working on what could be five out of your patient's six goals. Naturally, it isn't reasonable to have every single deficit acknowledged in each of the goals. Whatever you are working on explicitly, such as the improvement of memory or orientation, should be short- or long-term goals. Where you find the need to be a bit more general, you can leave the long-term goal to just outline, for example: "to facilitate improved-cognitive communication."

I must add that this doesn't mean your patient will be all set to solve a thousand-piece puzzle despite reaching all their cognitive goals. Even if you have a thousand-piece (or even a hundred-piece) puzzle and want to put into your goals that your patient will solve it, think again. For one, it's too hard for most people, even if they don't have an advanced cognitive problem. Second, it would never get done in your session time. Third, it's not a functional task, as the daily needs of the average adult do not require this specific skill.

Does that mean you can't use puzzles to work on your goals? Absolutely not. I strongly recommend it as an activity.

This being said, my advice for speech goals are:

- Don't look too far into the future.
- Avoid listing specific activities in the goals, unless it is an evidence-based exercise.
- Keep it functional.
- Keep it flexible.
- Drop what isn't working.

## ORDERS

Here you have to take some time to dissolve what you will really be treating.

Your patient who is post stroke, with several issues—which you have documented well in the write-up—may need attention for all of the modalities you service. Me, myself, and I—we have chosen that one person is too small and one 30-minute window is too narrow to achieve every miracle. Whatever you write in your orders reflects what you have documented as your diagnosis and that you have justified the patient's ability to participate in the treatment to improve the diagnosis.

### Speech

*ST Tx for (motor) speech 3-5x weekly for 4 weeks to facilitate improved intelligibility for communication with caregivers.*

This order means you have completed a comprehensive speech/language evaluation for the patient and, again, their function proved to be at least minimally decreased and a change from it was prior to their diagnosis. Remember that there are language differences and language disorders—the lines blur sometimes. Some people deal with having dysfluent speech or speaking less intelligibly for their entire lives. It is not ethical to place someone on therapy for an age-old speech problem, because their rehabilitation potential is significantly reduced. If they are communicating their needs well with nursing staff and are fairly intelligible, it's probably not worth the pick up, unless they request it.

This is matched with a diagnosis such as dysarthria or an acquired apraxia. While you can consider dysfluency, it is worth mentioning that this isn't the most effective phrasing; I would likely identify 'fluency' somewhere in there to specify.

### Language

*ST Tx for language 3-5x weekly for 4 weeks to facilitate improved expressive/receptive communication for improved function in ADLs.*

This order is matched with a diagnosis of aphasia or unspecified expressive or receptive deficits.

## Cognitive-communication

*ST Tx for cognitive-communication 3-5x weekly for 4 weeks to facilitate improved participation in ADLs.*

This order means you have completed a comprehensive speech/language evaluation for a patient's memory function, problem solving, and organization—and found it primarily impaired. Also included are decreased safety awareness, attention, and insight. These people require services because they are at greater risk of falls and other injurious behaviors.

This diagnosis has connections to various medical diagnoses. In your write-up, you will specify the treatment diagnosis as a cognitive-communication disorder. SLPs do not put dementia on the documentation, unless there is a dementia diagnosis already listed in the patient's case file.

One communicative modality is not all, and all are not the same. Take the time to reword the goals to include more than one modality when needed, and to generalize the purpose of the treatment, with the highlight always being to improve communication.

I would warn against writing an order for a speech or language-related modality for someone who is primarily being treated because of a cognitive-related issue, or vice versa. Someone who has altered mental status (AMS) may say the wrong month or day of the week, or call an item by the wrong name. It's likely due to cognition, and not an expressive language problem which is being exhibited as paraphasia. On the other hand, when someone has aphasia (with functional cognition) and says it is the month of September while it is the month of July, you can likely attribute it to the deficit in naming rather than a decreased orientation. It is truly a responsibility to weigh the evidence to form the correct interpretation of the person's difficulties.

An SLP may also choose to include both language and cognitive communication modalities if the evidence is not enough to distinguish between them. Based on the assessment, the patient has deficits in both areas, and the goals reflect this; therefore, so does the order. This is my usual approach.

Here is an example:

Once, when I saw a patient for what I supposed to be selective mutism, I focused on setting goals that were more cognitive than language-based (social communication, attention, and insight/awareness). Being that her disorder, schizophrenia, is entirely based on anxiety in certain social situations, her receptive and expressive communication should have been intact. When someone infrequently speaks, it's honestly difficult to get a good sample of evidence that they understand and can reply appropriately. In the times that I'd screened that patient and heard her speak, there were no concerns for anything aside from the fact that she rarely ever spoke to the staff. The diagnosis of schizophrenia was enough for me to decide on picking up for this particular purpose; however, I also wrote goals with receptive and expressive language in mind (responding to yes and no questions, and using two full sentences during a therapy session). This would be how I gauged the success of the cognitive approach on actual language production.

I'll be honest. It seemed like I had checked all my boxes and accounted for what I needed. However, it turned out that I approached this case a bit wrongly. The patient also had a diagnosis of dementia, and deficits in the receptive and expressive realms became clearer as time went by. The limited evidence base for selective mutism in adults and the role of the speech therapist was no help for me either. Because I had dual orders for speech-language and cognitive-communication intervention, I was able to transition my therapy to fit the patients needs as they were realized throughout the therapy course, although the true source of the problem was cloudy.

Sara Ipatenco, a published writer and teacher of health and nutrition, explains that in children, language development begets cognitive development[1]. When working with adults, it seems that what really begets improved overall function after a traumatic event (especially when language production has been affected) is cognitive rehabilitation. SLPs use an array of cognitive strategies to help patients relearn a language or skill. Richard Roberts and Roger Kreuz state in Becoming Fluent: How Cognitive Science Can Help Adults Learn a Foreign Language, "Adults shouldn't try to learn as children do; they should learn like adults."[2] While this text does not draw on language disability, it is agreeable in the sense that we can consider our patients to have some recollection or steadfastness to the way they know things should be done; that is to say—their social use of language and their knowledge of how language is used to get what they need.

# A Guide to the Voice Evaluation

Compared to swallow and cognitive-communication evaluations, the voice evaluation is quite rare in the long-term facility. I went about my chart review in the same way, but the referral process was different. I actually never got these types of referrals automatically—to be honest—I happened upon them by accident. This is how it worked for me: the patient would be a new admission whom I'd screened or was busy evaluating for some other problem. I talked to him or her to figure out just how long the problem had been persisting, and to get an overall idea of his or her view of the presenting deficits. I did not necessarily pick up right away, because most voice problems treat themselves or improve quickly as a patient rehabilitates. Note that diagnoses strongly related to voice loss, maybe multiple sclerosis or a tracheostomy, must be considered on an individual basis. To put it briefly, it really just depends. Remember that voice therapy is typically matched up with an ENT referral; if you plan to do voice therapy, you want to be in touch with the patient's physician to make sure it's possible. You also want to make sure that materials you'll need for your patient's continued improvement (e.g., a Passy-Muir Valve for a tracheostomy patient) are available to you at your facility. For these reasons, voice evaluations are far and few between. However, when it comes up, you want to be prepared for it.

## FIRST, THE CHART REVIEW

Because of the nature of the voice evaluation, the "chart review" is much more like the "patient review"—considering that many of the things you look for are many times not found directly in the chart, but instead through conversations with the patient and their family. Most of these will be 'in-house' or take place days to weeks beyond the initial evaluation (whether for speech/language or swallowing).

## Post-Acute

- Primary diagnosis and prior medical history.
- Prior level of functioning.
- Day-to-day activities.
- Medications.
- Nursing/Physician consultation.
- Family info.

## In-house

- Nursing note for some change in function (related to or aside from voice).
- Alertness of the patient and stimulability.
- Medication changes.
- New diagnoses.
- Patient interest and awareness of deficits.
- Insurance.
- Dependence on ventilator/trach.
- Participation in ADLs and social activities.

To touch on a few points:

All the diagnoses you will encounter often (that affect swallowing or speech/language) can be related to voice deficits, as well. It's not nearly as common, but there's no surprise—considering that respiration is our support for voicing, and nerve damage can affect motor function and sensation to the muscles most active in voicing.

Given that your patient is alert and somewhat oriented, you will get a chance to speak in depth with them. In the meantime, the chart may outline some vague details about their lives at home. If you know that they have eight hours or more in home health aide assistance, you can assume they don't spend a great deal of time talking to large groups or screaming across a classroom. Something that you might not find in the chart is that the patient is an avid football fan and spends each Thursday, Sunday, and Monday screaming at a television.

Medications may play some part in vocal changes, but a quick conversation with the nurse or physician will clear that up quite easily.

The second best person to speak to, other than the patient, would be a family member who knows how they usually sound and can help you form a distinction and timeline, to help you understand the patient's needs better.

With an in-house patient, you'll not usually receive a note specific to voice; instead the nurse may generalize it to a 'new speech problem.' In either case, your documentation will outline what you noticed and why you went ahead with a voice evaluation. We set aside voice therapy for people who are stable, alert, able to follow directions, and genuinely care about improving their status. It will not be successful in most other cases, especially with passive techniques. Because an ENT will be on your referral list 99.9% of the time during this therapy course, you want to be aware of whether the patient's insurance can cover them for this. As they say... "Healthcare ain't cheap!"

If the patient can see an ENT to rule out a physical vocal pathology, you can hit the track running. Of course, if there is any physical vocal pathology, you want to talk to the physician about the usefulness of voice therapy prior to any needed surgery.

## GATHER YOUR MATERIALS

- Voice evaluation template.
- Penlight.
- Straw.
- Tissue.
- Timer.
- Sound level meter.
- Dry spirometer (forced vital capacity).
- Reading passage.

Note: I won't get into all the state-of-the-art voice programs, such as The Multidimensional Voice Program and CSL-Pitch program, because I don't know that they are accessible in this setting. They were not accessible for me, but from information gathered, I've learned that they also take very long to administer, which is not ideal for the SNF setting. In a clinic, they may allot you more time and greater access to those materials. In the SNF, the mantra is: more work in less time.

Feel free to use mobile apps when they're available. I learned about free apps from YouTube videos, one of them being VoiceTest, which measures an estimate of voice shimmer and jitter. You may find this useful for your patient.

## THE ASSESSMENT

Thankfully, the voice assessment is not as time consuming as the speech-language or even dysphagia evaluation can be. It is quite straightforward; after checking off a few boxes, the evaluation is pretty much complete. You can choose to take extra time to record a speech sample (with the patient's permission) to assess how his or her voice changes over time properly. Listening to someone speak is like watching paint dry—not in the sense of it being boring, but in the sense that you might not notice subtle things that occur over several seconds or minutes.

Start the evaluation with a thorough patient interview. Ask questions about their everyday routine and their experience with the use of their voice. This is the only way you can provide useful recommendations and sound therapeutic intervention. If they never drink water, this is something you should be aware of and monitor for improvements over time. If they have always spoken in a whisper, you shouldn't attempt to turn them into a peewee league football coach.

Motor speech components are crucial to check during the voice evaluation, as it helps to distinguish a potential dual disorder or concomitant deficit that complicates the original problem. An example is an oral resonance problem that occurs after an adequate vocal vibration. Perhaps prosody can be considered, which explains why a patient might enter and prolong vocal fry in the middle of a sentence with no real need to be based on vocal pathology. As the evaluator, you may use models to cue the desired outcome; however, the success of these may depend on the overall view of the patient.

Don't bother giving the patient additional opportunities to complete a task, hoping they will do better with subsequent attempts. If anything, their voice is wearing out with each new task you give. Doing fifteen attempts for sustained phonation can decrease their energy for doing ten s/z ratios. The first one or two are likely the best they can do, and breaks in between the tasks may help.

Whatever supplemental oxygen being provided should remain exactly as indicated by the orders, and you should document it. Obviously, with respiratory deficits, the individual is at a disadvantage for performance in the evaluation.

## GOAL WRITING

Again, the voice modality of our field is really straightforward. Your goals should be specific and measurable. Compared to dysphagia and speech goals, you will not resort to mostly subjective means to measure success after the initial evaluation. When working on dysphagia and speech goals, you are seeing the patient in a variety of situations, discussing various topics, or watching them eat various types of meals, with the consistency/texture and bolus size changing slightly with each bite. With voice, you can literally measure the patient's decibel level with a free app on your cell phone.

That being said, your goals should initially reflect some sort of numerical value that you're using to track your patient's progress.

Here is an example:

*Patient will increase sustained phonation to ___ seconds, using moderate cues to apply diaphragmatic breathing technique, to facilitate improved volume during speaking tasks.*

*Patient will tolerate Passy-Muir valve for ___ minutes with close ST supervision during therapy session to increase ability to manage respiration for speaking.*

You won't be straying too far from exactly what your evaluation tasks were. These will directly influence the patient's vocal abilities. Contrarily, for the dysphagia and speech evaluations, you will typically do only 1/10 of the tasks you try to incorporate during the therapy. Of course, as the patient progresses, you will incorporate more complex tasks like speaking over a loud television or singing a song without losing volume or having voice breaks. You may immediately recommend some vocal hygiene or implement them as strategies, such as increasing the patient's water intake.

## ORDERS

*ST Tx for 3-5x weekly for 4 weeks to facilitate improved vocal clarity and volume for communication during ADLs.*

You can reword the order as needed, such as if your patient has a tracheostomy and the goal is to implement the use of a Passy-Muir valve.

# A Guide to the Write-Up, Notes, and Discharge

I briefly covered documentation for dysphagia evaluations, but here are a few more pointers:

- Connect the dots by outlining the evaluation from beginning to end.
- Don't just use the 'build' functions on your EMR; notate and explain where necessary, and summarize.
- Use as many objective markers as possible (e.g., amount of seconds, number of successful attempts, etc.).
- Specify changes you have noticed over time that could complicate the severity level or ability to complete a task (e.g., if the patient had mild difficulty at the beginning which progressed to moderate later on).

Once you have written your documentation, outlined the details of the evaluation, made a treatment diagnosis, set your goals, and made your recommendations... what happens next?

A typical turnover for therapy is 28 days. This does not mean you need all that time, nor that it's enough. It is a standard square of time used to establish the therapy course. You can cut it short or extend it as you see fit. The record of progress during this course of time will include daily treatment encounter notes and progress notes. At the end of the 28 days, if you feel like the therapy course should continue, you will write a recertification.

The short-term objectives should be discussed in each note you write for the patient. With as much detail as possible, cover what the patient's response to the activities has been, whether the patient has made any progress, what your plans are to continue the course of therapy, and why. Justifying only necessary therapy is key to maintaining our ethics as healthcare professionals.

When the patient meets all his or her goals or reaches a plateau and cannot surpass a certain level of achievement, therapy is no longer needed, and it is time to discharge. Discharge documentation should be just as clearly and carefully worded as the evaluation and the recertification (if you've made one). Long- and short-term goals are addressed as completely as possible. Recommendations are essentially final until there arises some need for another pick up of this patient, so some regard to training caregivers and staff should be taken.

As you may know, the SNF is a place of unexpected happenings. An unplanned discharge may occur for a patient who has been hospitalized. Further, a patient may experience a steep decline that no longer warrants a rehabilitative approach. This may mean comfort care or hospice care, which we'll talk about in We've Come this Far by Faith (chapter 15). Our most likely concern upon reaching this point is the patient's swallow function. If the patient can consume any oral intake, an appropriate diet consistency and set of precautions should be outlined and caregivers should be trained and observed carefully with techniques. The medical team will be extensively involved in a case like this, and communication with them will be critical. Discharges upon time of expiration—that is, when the patient has passed away—will be detailed to summarize the therapy course leading up to the unplanned event.

**CHAPTER FOOTNOTES**

[1]Ipatenco, Sara "How Does Language Development Affect Cognitive Development?" How To Adult, April 18, 1970. https://howtoadult.com/language-development-affect-cognitive-development-6388730.html.

[2]Roberts, Richard, and Roger J. Kreuz. Becoming Fluent: How Cognitive Science Can Help Adults Learn a Foreign Language. Cambridge, MA: The MIT Press, 2016.

# 10

# DO I HAVE TO CALL?

*A Guide to the Referral Process*

It sounds like an old 90s R&B song, but it's really the millions of call bells going off in your head as you realize your patient's problems are beyond what you are equipped to handle.

A part of working with complex patients is knowing how to access different levels and areas of their care and the right times to do so. In the SNF, you may have limited reach to all the other kinds of professionals one patient may need. You can reach out to the primary medical provider for any reason. He or she will be present at the facility at least a few days a week. However, when it's not urgent or does not require word-of-mouth permission to write an order, even those doctors can be a bit bothered by your phone call. Nursing supervisors are usually your best bet to understand how to proceed with your referral. Even if you already have the answers, a quick note to them will at least leave them in the know. After all, they are primarily responsible for the patients on their respective units.

## THE WHY
*Referral Checklist*

Ten ways to know you need to talk to another professional to do your job fully:

1. You sense that a patient's problems with speech, language, or swallowing fall outside the realm of the physical mouth and pharynx and have not yet been diagnosed. Example: If the problem seems to be nasal, laryngeal (at the level of or below the vocal cords), esophageal (after the completion of the swallow), cognitive (with no diagnosis of dementia or known medical problem related to cognitive decline), or related to a new medication, you must speak with the nursing supervisor to get a better understanding of the situation. He or she will then take the lead to confer with the doctor.

2. Your provision of a service, especially dysphagia therapy, is contraindicated by another diagnosis (e.g., esophageal or gastrointestinal disorder).

3. Your patient has been in a state of functioning that requires the use of an assistive device

(e.g., a PEG tube) for a long time, and you seek to change or alter the demand for it.
4. You need an objective test.
5. Your patient is declining while you are providing rehabilitative services.
6. Your patient is sick or complains of physical distress during any session.
7. Your patient increasingly exhibits emotional distress, or uses negative or abusive speech.
8. Your patient is improving in skills unrelated to your services.
9. Your recommendations are not being carried out adequately (by the patient, staff, or family members).
10. Your therapy is not working, and the patient is still at significant risk of aspiration, weight loss, or other complications.

## THE HOW
*Approaching Your Fellow Professionals*

As the chapter title indicates, referring is not always easy. It's not scheduled into your day, so there goes a blemish onto your productivity. It's quite hard to locate people in the building. Phones ring off the hook, and messages don't always get delivered. Not to mention, your co-workers are always busy, even if they're on break. You take it or you leave it. Sometimes you have those people who are good listeners, even when they're juggling a million things. Some others forget what you said as soon as you leave the room. The best you can do is to be attentive and sensitive—within reasonable boundaries. When it's not a good time to share loads of important information, it's easier to just come back later, rather than to repeat it on six other occasions.

It would, of course, help to gauge the level of urgency the problem holds for your patient. Some referrals are best held off for a few days after initially noticing a problem. People are more receptive to observations with some broad basis. If you are forgetful, I recommend that you always write things down so you can provide a wealth of detail to support your general idea. In a more urgent situation, repetitively reporting to a person can get them on their feet and moving. Honestly, many times after you refer, you will have to do some level of follow-up. That being said, you will also want to gauge the responsiveness of the professional you are dealing with.

Remember that people count on you to be responsive as well. Often, CNAs came to me directly to speak about patients, rather than taking their concerns to the nursing supervisors, just because they knew me well and had a grasp on what I could offer within my scope. While it complicates the intended chain of referral, I would usually screen the patient before or after speaking to the nursing supervisor. If the nursing supervisor is unaware of the patient's changed behavior, it will benefit you to go to the patient beforehand, as realistically, the nursing supervisor won't pose a great help to you if you asked them specific questions.

## JUMPING THE OBSTACLES
*Dealing with Not-So-Helpful Co-workers*

While the focus of this chapter is not about managing relationships in the building (I already did that in chapter 5—The New Guy on the Block), I want to reiterate that learning to communicate effectively in your workplace will be key to getting what you want. It sounds absurd, because it's not even a favor on your part; you're really advocating for another human, for whom your fellow professionals are also responsible. The fact, however, is that people would be more adamant about making sure you get a piece of cake at a staff party than making sure they go to see a patient you told them is begging for their attention. Still, their view of what's right and what's necessary might not align with yours. So, however you see it, you really have to pitch it. Co-workers who are willing to listen are the ones who respect and like you. That's the indecent way the cookie crumbles.

There will be people you must use as a referral point who are just difficult to speak to. I mentioned earlier my poor relationship with the primary doctor at my facility. Really, he was one of the rudest, most diminutive people I had ever met. Simply greeting him in the halls became tasking, and I intentionally reduced our contact to a point of speaking only when spoken to and when necessary. Well, 'necessary' turned out to be at least once a week. So, once a week, I mustered up the courage to keep a straight face with unfurled eyebrows and do what had to be done.

My memory clearly portrays my feet dragging step by step through the halls, knowing I had to make a phone call to this doctor for an MBS referral. The golden standard video fluoroscopic swallow study, known also as the modified barium swallow, was the second most difficult type of referral in all of my time in a SNF. The most difficult one was an ENT consult I attempted for a tracheostomy patient who could potentially have been a candidate for a Passy-Muir valve for speaking. This request was shot down in seconds, then revived long enough for me to make about five more stops to build some back-up (I had the rehab director on my side, as well as my supervisor and the nursing supervisor). Our army was weak, and we all fell. With practice, one becomes more prepared for these conversations when equipped with a supportive defense, text evidence, and near-trivia knowledge about the patient's profile. It helps to accustom yourself to hearing "no", so you're never short of the energy to negotiate or at least ask, "why not?". It should always be documented that you tried to obtain the help of an outside service and what the outcome was.

"Do I Have to Call?" can also lend itself to 'telling' or 'relaying' information for the sake of your patients or your quality of work. I've had to turn up the heat a little at times, because even after doing my part, speaking to the appropriate caregivers and professionals, and clearly documenting my recommendation, they did not follow through.

It's your duty to push it to the limit. Your referral process is your responsibility to your patients to ensure the highest level of quality care for them, which is never something you can do all by yourself. You can't just ignore it or forget about it when people are terrible listeners. Your reputation, your license, and your patient are all on the line.

So how do you make all of it go a bit smoother?

Just slightly tangential to referring is in-servicing. In an in-service, you're giving out needed bits of information about what you do, why you do it, and how to apply what you share. Essentially, you are leading a group training, and the goal is to have people walk away more informed and, hopefully, able to sensibly utilize what was discussed.

The key in in-servicing is that everyone is away from their other responsibilities, able to more adequately focus on what you're saying. Most often, they have to complete a quiz or sign off on having been present and learning this information. With their signature they agree to comply, so this is a bit more concrete than passive word-of-mouth, although you should make sure to document that, too.

## STORY TIME WITH RENA
### Thermal Stimulation

Rena's story reflects many of the points I make in We've Come This Far by Faith (chapter 15).

Considering her family's stance on only providing what was absolutely necessary for her to be comfortable, Rena was never allowed a feeding tube, despite her dysphagia problem being extremely severe. I didn't form much resistance on the point; instead, I did everything I could think of to make her problem less severe and trained the staff and family to respond to it more adequately. The only thing that seemed to work was a metal spoon chilled in ice. Eventually, she received these spoons at every meal, but most often, the staff did not even use them. She coughed and coughed as the CNAs continued to feed her. I came to a point of lividity when I realized how shamelessly people I had pretty good working relationships with simply ignored my training and recommendations. I heard every excuse in the book, but it came down to successive conversations with higher-ups to ensure the reinforcement of the recommendations.

All over a damn spoon.

# 11

# NOW LET'S GET LITERATE

## *A Guide on How to Write Clinically*

The next, biggest part of your job—yes, still bigger than your therapy in the eyes of the 'man'—is your paperwork. A popular saying is, "If it's not written down, it didn't happen."

You ask, "So, if it is written down, it did! Right?" Well, not if it really didn't.

Treat your paperwork as though you will defend it in a court of law. You may never see this actually happen, but the reality is that your paperwork is a binding contract—you do what you say you will. You enforce your recommendations like a squad car pulling them over for doing 85 in a 50, and you write that ticket every time:

*'Nursing staff re-educated on diet and safety precautions. Will follow up.'*

On a serious note, never write down something that didn't happen. It will bite you right in the ass. Consider that what you report may strongly mis-align with what several other professionals in the building are writing or saying, and that's a no-no. Creative phrasing is everything in documentation, but do not ever lie.

The first thing you want to know about your paperwork is whether it is digital or paper-based. If it is purely paper-based, you are almost guaranteed to hate your job. However, you're quite lucky if it is digital. It seems that most facilities these days use a mix of both. The facilities I worked at maintained paper charts; while orders, nursing notes, and all rehab documentation were recorded through EMRs (Electronic Medical Records). It takes some getting used to, but the quickness of EMRs make productivity much more achievable and mistakes easy to correct, though, of course, we want to do our best to be accurate the first time around. You will—before long—get a handle of the quick selections to build your segments, and treatment notes and progress notes will be done in five minutes at most.

I'll get to how you can write creatively as a clinician later in this chapter, and I've already touched on the specifics for evaluations and orders in Tidbits (chapter 9, but here I want to expand a bit further on how paperwork really makes the nursing rehab world go 'round.

## NO JUSTICE WITHOUT JUSTIFICATION

PEG (percutaneous endoscopic gastronomy) tube, otherwise known as G-tube or enteral feeding, is a great area to explore to understand how important documentation is. Because it's long-term, often for the remainder of the patient's life span, you'll do some of your best creative writing around these cases. One thing we have to consider is the amount of money it costs to guarantee something for the rest of someone's life. With that, we can appreciate why insurance companies regularly check in to make sure their money is wisely used. They don't just check the one time the patient had, say, a stroke, and let that be the end-all, be-all into the unforeseeable future. In fact, foreseeable futures are the only thing we, as a medical community, can count on. When documenting for a PEG tube patient, you are utilizing regular screening(yearly, or more frequently) and making at least some attempts at engaging the patient in rehabilitative care. Taking this case by case, you'll find some patients who can eat a little bit, but not a full meal. Others may tolerate a meal. With some, you'll have regular therapy, hopeful for a full transition to PO (oral) feeding, while others will have a specified amount for pleasure feeding by mouth. No matter what they or you do, if these patients still get their primary or even supplemental nutrition from the PEG tube, justification will be necessary. The dietician will offer you invaluable help in these cases; but when you document, you must give the viewpoint from your scope. This has to be outlined specifically, without any room for misconception.

You'll want to start by identifying a related diagnosis. Failure to thrive, severe dysphagia, and esophageal dysmotility may all suffice. Dementia, in the absence of a functional swallowing difficulty, is not sufficient for the justification of a PEG tube. How then do you respond when a dementia patient chooses not to eat more than three bites of their meal, or only wants ice cream? It becomes complex, and these situations have to be taken case by case. You'll be, at times, overextended for cases like these because the dietician has likely tried some sort of adjustment to enhance caloric intake, but ruling out or confirming a dysphagia is one of the many steps taken along the way to the PEG tube placement.

First, you try everything within your power of encouragement and magic. Dementia is a peculiar diagnosis, and it comes in so many shapes and colors. Sometimes you can get through with some sensory or thermal stimulation. Given the situation, you can try turning all the food into liquids; if the person will drink, it can be helpful. You could try changing the environment or the look of the food within reasonable boundaries and ability. If that fails, it only leaves you with your findings; and hopefully, the patient is left with Ensure. Ensure truly saves lives. The dietician will probably be on top of supplements before you even have a chance to blink, but keep him or her updated on what you notice during your course of therapy.

Speaking of therapy, I have to be honest. Justification for this kind of therapy is somewhat... airy. It's not a dysphagia, though some may highlight the decreased 'oral acceptance' as an 'oral dysphagia.' We'll agree to disagree. Yes, it's still defendable in a court of law, as the SLP holds a wealth of knowledge of ways to intervene, and certainly there's the need to do something before the situation becomes as severe as a failure to thrive or an acquired dysphagia. It's a routine measure that I support, though it's rarely been successful and quite frustrating in my experience. You'll get more info in your survival guide on dementia (see Chapter 14), but for now, documenting everything you've tried is the best you can offer.

This all being said, I made the mistake once of highlighting dementia in a case in which the patient was receiving PEG tube feeding over a long period, but who was a candidate for pleasure feeding. She was doing great—taking part in exercises and eating lots of pudding. She had some gastric issues aside from a behavioral-cognitive deficit, but dysphagia wasn't really a primary problem anymore. Looking back on her old paperwork, 'severe dysphagia' was documented. I didn't know her all the way back then; perhaps she'd magically gotten better—it happens. However, there's never too little room to have the passing thought of how many healthcare professionals exaggerate or even lie to please insurance companies.

The patient's insurance refused to cover her enteral feeding for at least a month after I commented on her feeding problem being primarily cognitive. Everyone, as you can assume, was ready to kill me. The situation was rectified, and not because I followed suit and exaggerated a miniscule problem. There are plenty of ways to otherwise strongly document your view and convince your audience, who is—in this case—Showtime at Medicaid, featuring Jevity and 45 Degrees. It'll either be a standing ovation or you'll be booed to the stage exit.

## MORE THAN JUST WORDS

In my and perhaps any medical SLP's experience—the way I've phrased things in my documentation has meant the difference between extending or immediately ending therapy, receiving PEG tube feeding or having PO feeding, insurance coverage or non-coverage, and many more possibilities. I would not say that it has truly meant the difference between life and death, but as I'll discuss in Mom and Pop (chapter 16), we are made to make careful decisions when a patient is approaching the end of the road. Otherwise, the doctors and nurses are more consistently and holistically aware of the patient, and will make emergency decisions when needed. As long as we document sensibly, they can appreciate our part in caring for the patient.

Sometimes, it's no extreme situation. Especially in long-term care, we have patients who cannot function well enough in the therapy to achieve success. A patient who is confused, distracted, unmotivated, or simply tired may be someone that doesn't make too many gains right away. With these patients, you want to be selective and carefully evaluate the source of the problem and ways to overcome it.

If a patient doesn't participate in therapy for a week, and you suspect it may be a new medication that they're on that's causing the problem, take time to talk to the nurses and see what can be done to mitigate its effects. Otherwise, just your part in documenting and communicating.

While you're doing your fair share, be sure that your documentation is easy to understand for the layman. Consider that people from other health professions are laymen in yours. Keep it concise but informative. I suggest using fewer abbreviations, especially if they aren't common, and even more so if you're notating on an EMR. It's not as cool in the new technology era and really doesn't save that much time, anyway.

Take care of how you speak about your patients. There is no excuse for speaking about a patient in a way that is diminutive or rude. Be equally considerate with your co-workers. Remember, these documents are around for a long time. Your documentation represents you, so write in a way that conveys what you want others to perceive.

| INSTEAD OF: | SAY THIS: |
|---|---|
| Patient doesn't like me and won't do my exercises. | The patient frequently turns away from the ST when prompted to participate in lingual exercises. Patient has frequently become agitated and verbally aggressive. Not typically responsive to redirection or encouragement, resulting in discontinuation of exercises. |
| Patient is belligerent and won't make any more progress. | The patient frequently screams and exercises physically and verbally violent behaviors. Due to noted aggressiveness, the patient is not considerably a good candidate for continued intervention, as this presents a harm to the patient and ST. Recommended that nursing re-refer if any changes. |
| Patient's family is completely insusceptible to new information. | Patient and caregivers/family have been repeatedly educated on safety precautions, diet texture, and compensatory strategies. Carry-over has been poor, despite explicit instruction. Nursing supervisor has been notified of family's attempts to feed patient items from advanced diet consistency, and has verbalized plan to follow up with family. |

| | |
|---|---|
| Patient is completely insusceptible to new information. | Patient has received maximal assistance and multimodal cueing to achieve <25% success with compensatory strategy. No functional carry-over has been noted, rendering the need for a discontinuation of training procedures. Staff should continue to anticipate all needs, using recommended strategies as educated. |
| Patient wants but does not need a diet upgrade (Soon after being seen for therapy.) | Patient has been noted with frequent requests for food items from an advanced diet consistency. Patient most recently seen 1/3/2020–1/15/2020 for dysphagia therapy, and was unable to meet long term goals, despite improving tolerance of nectar-thick liquids. Achieved upgrade to nectar-thick liquids prior to d/c of ST program. At this time, patient does not warrant continued therapy intervention due to decreased ability to cooperate and follow directives during oral and pharyngeal exercise. Additionally, patient is edentulous and does not wear dentures, which was noted to increase difficulty during mastication. It is recommended that patient continue on current diet consistency (puree + nectar-thick liquids). |
| Patient takes too long to eat solid food. None of the CNAs are as patient as I am to take 30+ minutes per meal. | Patient has been assisted during meal time, during which the patient trialed chopped solids. Due to moderately prolonged mastication with additional measures taken to facilitate oral clearance (i.e. alternation of bites/sips), patient takes a total of 30+ minutes to consume meal in its entirety. To reduce patient and caregiver burden, as well as to reduce risks related to fatigue during meal, it is recommended that patient continue on softer consistency (i.e. puree). |

| | |
|---|---|
| Patient has too many other things going on. Come back when you have all your stuff together. | Patient has been seen for screening, after consult from nursing for noted difficulty with communication and orientation. Patient is currently consuming puree + nectar-thick liquid diet consistency and tolerating well with good PO intake. The patient, however, presents as extremely lethargic after readmission from acute hospitalization 3 days ago. Nursing has communicated that patient is receiving additional medication to manage symptoms, which is suspected to contribute to patients' overall mental status. Patient is not a candidate for ST intervention at this time, as prognosis for improvement is poor, due to the patient's decreased ability to remain alert for session time and follow directions. Re-refer given increased alertness and continued deficits in cognitive-communication. |
| Patient can't focus for three seconds to imitate a model. | Patient has exhibited moderate-maximal difficulty attending to models, and has been unable to imitate given 10 opportunities during session time. |

| | |
|---|---|
| Patient coughs all day long, I don't think they're coughing during meals because of food, but I can't prove it because I can't get an MBS. | Patient has been noted with baseline cough throughout course of therapy. Cough suppressant has been prescribed, per communication with nursing. Coughing intermittently during meals; however, this does not typically occur immediately after the swallow. Coughing is dry and non-productive. Patient exhibits improvements in bolus control, swallow timing, and hyolaryngeal elevation. When asked, patient communicates having no discomfort with food consistency. At this time, patient is recommended to continue this diet consistency, with close supervision. Notify nursing supervisor and ST if coughing increases in frequency or presents with wet quality during the meal. |

In these notes, when possible and appropriate I have:

- Drawn attention to what kind of service was provided, and why.
- Included subjective and objective points.
- Outlined specifics about the number of attempts, success rate, situation and changes and modifications provided.
- Made diet consistency clear, as to never be guessed.
- Not put anyone down with my language.
- Outlined my response to a problem, even if it didn't work.
- Stayed on topic.
- Not shown any personal response, even if I did take it personally.
- Outlined communication with other professionals.
- Mentioned any prior attempts to achieve something, dates, and why it didn't work.
- Made recommendations.
- Provided intentions for follow-up.

What you may see is more words, and I do have a history of being wordy. It helps me understand and remember better what exactly occurred, and if someone else is covering my caseload, I don't have to be concerned that they don't have enough information to go forward.

Since we, as rehab therapists, are technically not paid for documentation—therefore requiring you to fit it into a small square of allotted "non-productive" time, I would recommend any less wordy way you find to make your documentation clear. While it's a balancing act of sorts, I trust that your fingers will move much faster, and that your thought process will be much tidier by the end of your CFY than at the beginning.

# 12

# CHA-CHING!

## *A Guide to Billing*

After all is said and done, it's time to balance the books—I mean, the insurance company. Billing is easily the most important task of your day, but also the quickest. It gets the facility paid and ultimately gets you paid. You must do this before you leave the building, and round it to the nearest five minutes. Most often, your sessions will last 30 minutes. Billing for 30 minutes is acceptable if you use the last five minutes to write notes or train staff. However, it is not acceptable if your patient spent five minutes sleeping, five minutes refusing to participate, and five minutes heading to the bathroom.

While billing is straightforward, there is a lot running in the background with your rehab director driving your department's contribution to the facility's money. You won't really be active in that area, so let him or her handle the math. Do your part to be responsible and ethical by reporting only the minutes that you feel are owed for your time and effort.

## CPT CODES

Here's what we generally see and think about when it comes to billing:

| SERVICE/ MODALITY | TYPE | CPT CODE |
|---|---|---|
| Speech-Language / Voice | Evaluation | 92506 |
| Speech-Language/ Voice | Therapy | 92507 |
| Speech-Language | Group Therapy | 92508 |
| Dysphagia | Evaluation | 92610 |
| Dysphagia | Therapy | 92526 |
| Cognition (primary) | Evaluation | 96125 |
| Cognition (primary) | Therapy | 97129 |

*G0515 was recently used prior to implementation of 97129, and discontinued on January 1, 2020.

| MINUTES (PER DAY) | CONCURRENT ALLOWANCE | STANDARDIZED |
|---|---|---|
| 60 | NO | NO |
| 30 | YES | |
| 30 | NO | |
| 60 | NO | NO |
| 30 | YES | |
| 60 | NO | YES |
| 15 | YES | |

These minutes may change with the notice of your rehab director. For instance, she or he may assign additional minutes to a session to meet minute requirements before the patient's assessment reference date. You may also request more time in your schedule to work on a more time-consuming activity with a patient or to help them realize some success if the 30 minutes regularly proves to be too little for them.

Evaluation includes the time you take to complete a chart review, assess the patient, confer with the nursing staff, and write your notes. Where you see 60 minutes, the billing will actually reflect 30 minutes designated to the 'treatment' of the patient and the other 30 minutes to the 'actual' evaluation. Your evaluation may take especially long for a variety of reasons. For example, a dysphagia evaluation may be extended if, after several consistency trials, none appear to be safe for the patient and additional measures and consultations need to be made. If it is a dual evaluation for both speech-language and swallowing, it would obviously take more time. I typically billed additional minutes whenever speech-language was considered. Compared to a dysphagia evaluation, it's almost impossible to do all the above in 60 minutes.

Treatment for any modality—consider speech-language to be interchangeable with cognitive-communication or voice—will yield the same amount of total time for treatment for one day, unless otherwise discussed or mandated. You may have to split your daily session minutes if more than one modality receives attention during the course of therapy. For instance, if you have a patient with a dysphagia diagnosis and dysarthria, you can place 15 minutes into the dysphagia service and 15 minutes into the speech-language service. Note that you must apply a minimum of eight minutes to each service billed for each day.

Each modality has a current procedural terminology (CPT) code that will guide the reimbursement owed for the treatment you provide. While I have outlined therapy for cognition, the American Speech-Language-Hearing Association (ASHA) recommends that you still use a speech-language CPT code if the intervention is not primarily cognitive. Have a detailed discussion about this with your supervisor and rehab director to ensure that you apply the correct codes to the documentation.

I use the 92506 and 92507 codes (speech-language or cognitive-communication evaluation and therapy respectively) as opposed to 96125 and 97129 (primary cognitive evaluation and therapy)—which caters for several professional perspectives, such as behavioral therapy—because the initial two are relative and specific to our scope. Many other professionals use a similar activity base with the goal of helping the patient to increase neuroplasticity and to become more involved and independent in their daily activities. Speech-language and primary cognitive intervention codes cannot be combined for use on the same day, and it is most sensible to use a speech-related code as an SLP.

At times, I've scurried my way to the floors at 10:30 just to see what the activities staff were working on for that day. Whether it was a trivia game or Hangman, if I had a patient who needed to improve in cognitive-communication or even speech and language, especially if a social component was a part of the patient's goals, it was a good opportunity to get them involved. Doing this is billable, and, of course, your contribution is to encourage the patient to participate and provide cues to increase their probability of success.

Whenever I saw that a patient had a bit of an attention or memory deficit, or whatever led me to believe he or she was a candidate for communication therapy, I provided a fairly broad assessment, compared to a standardized battery. When I provided this assessment, I attempted to rule out receptive and expressive language deficits and oral motor deficits, but these are more often than not affected as a result of the cognitive problem. When I created my goals, they were always cognitive and language based. For this reason, I billed 92506. I would not have ever found myself in the position to bill for a primarily cognitive approach, because it would have inhibited me from providing a language intervention. (The code 96125 indicates that language was either not tested, or that it wasn't included in the overall view of the patient's deficits). I also indicated that I used a standardized approach, which is unusual in the SNF setting. Third, the treatment code associated with this only covers 15 minutes of intervention—not 30. To work for a full 30 minutes on 'cognitive therapy,' one must bill under code 97130 for an additional 15 minutes.

The way I understand it from ASHA's website, CPT codes underwent a change in 2014 to divide the activities that all fell under the same umbrella code 92506, which was designated for all evaluations related to speech, language, voice, and communication. Depending on the facility, the CPT codes that you use might reflect the newer, 'broken-down' codes or that of the umbrella code.

| DIAGNOSTIC ASSESSMENT | CPT CODE | TREATMENT INDICATION/ CODE |
|---|---|---|
| Speech Fluency | 92521 | 92507 |
| Speech Sound | 92522 | 92507 |
| Speech Sound with expressive/ receptive language assessment* | 92523 | 92507 |
| Voice and Resonance | 92524 | 92507 |

*G0515 was recently used prior to implementation of 97129, and discontinued on January 1, 2020.

Personally, I don't think it makes a difference what your facility decides. Its only real purpose is to reimburse the SLP for providing intervention on different disorders as compared to just one. If the time is accounted for correctly, you can bill for your full contribution. Again, a conversation with your rehab director will clear this up quickly.

Where you see 'concurrent allowance' in the first table, I indicate here that there is no possibility to evaluate two patients at once; however, you may treat two patients at once, given the notice of your rehab director, which will reflect the allowance for such a service by the insurance. Generally, Medicare Part A and Medicaid patients may receive concurrent treatment, while Medicare Part B does not allow for this at all. Concurrent therapy suggests that there is some overlap in the time that patients are being treated, and that they are not working on the same activity or modality. Your EMR will have a section for you to plug in the overlap time, as it may not be the full length of the 30-minute session. It then automatically applies your actual time worked, considering that you were working with more than one patient. I never treated concurrently in the SNF. The two times that I did were the most complicated billing had ever been; but even then, it isn't something that takes more than one try to get down pat.

Group therapy is being encouraged more and more in the SNF setting, therefore you will be able to bill for 2–6 patients for therapy for the same or similar activity. This amounts to a total time of four hours if, for example, you see a group of four members for an entire hour of therapy. Can you guess why it is being encouraged more in this setting? That's right: 'more money, less time,' is the motto. Anyway, group and concurrent therapy are both limited to 25% of total therapy provision under the Patient-Driven Payment Model (PDPM), which we'll talk about more later (see chapter 13—PDPM).

## G-Codes

I'm not at all an expert in G-codes, since my facility only required the use of them for a short amount of time after I started working there. They were set aside for Medicare Part B patients; their purpose was to specify the functional limitation and severity at the initiation and end of therapy and the goal status for the therapy. Though they are no longer mandatory, a quick review is helpful.

ASHA has a long list of digital EMRs on their website. I don't know how to use a single one of them. I have been trained with Optima Healthcare Solutions—otherwise known as Rehab Optima—and using it for billing is straightforward and simple for me. Despite some horrible reviews from users who have apparently experienced something better, faster, and more reliable, Rehab Optima gets the job done, in my opinion. It is cloud based and can be used anywhere that has an internet connection. It is also cheaper than other similar systems, so perhaps this explains why it is a common nursing-household name. I don't know of any facility that still uses a stone-age paper billing system. If you don't use EMR for anything else, I believe at least the billing will be digital. Whatever your situation, ensure that this part of the day is quick and simple. You'll have to be a pro at it almost immediately.

## THE PROCESS

Whether you are using the Optima platform or another EMR, there should be an option to access patient assignments for the day. You'll see the minutes scheduled, CPT codes assigned from evaluation documentation, options to add additional billing codes, and options to add treatment encounter notes (TEN). Your facility will determine the requirements for TENs, so consult with your rehab director about the need for these. On the billing document, you'll also see an option to use concurrent treatment minutes, which you simply leave empty if you saw your patient individually.

## Missed treatment

Patients who are not seen for the day or seen for a decreased number of minutes of therapy on a day that they are scheduled—especially if this occurs for consecutive days—may later have a shortage of minutes leading up to their assessment reference date (ARD). Don't be alarmed if you make up for this time in following sessions, which may become 45 minutes instead of 30. If a patient misses the session altogether, a reason should be documented; this may include patient sickness, medical hold, transfer to hospital or a doctor's appointment, or simply a refusal to participate.

## Billable vs. Non-Billable

Remember, you can only bill for what you provide. Therefore, if a patient has an objective test like the modified barium swallow (CPT code 92610), you would not place minutes onto your billing document for it, as this is likely not a service you will provide.

Contrarily, you may bill minutes for any face-to-face interaction with your patient that relates to their goals. Having lunch across the table from your patient while chatting about astrology is lovely, but not billable. Your patient's goals are pursued by skilled instruction through techniques and strategies, caregiver involvement and education, and relevant activities or exercises. If you can justify that engaging with your patient in activities related to speech-language or swallowing was to their benefit, it just might be billable.

Non-billable (also known as non-patient care) time may be recorded in the EMR to account for time spent in the facility without being face-to-face with a patient. This can include purposes such as in-service, documentation, or meetings. Even transporting patients or assisting other staff members can be recorded. Other miscellaneous things come up during the day, but to protect your productivity percentages, you want to be mindful about keeping these things as minimally time-consuming as possible.

## Corrections and E-signing

As with all documentation, billing should be reviewed carefully prior to submitting it. Making corrections on an EMR is much simpler than with paper documents. When a patient is billed, the rehab director makes adjustments to the remainder of the patient's planned care. If you billed the patient for the wrong amount of minutes, recalculations can be an inconvenience. I have also found that you lose access to billing documents after a month. Corrections require extra permissions in such cases. Make sure that the original and corrected versions of any document are signed and dated on the EMR.

# 13

# PDPM

## A Guide to Ever-Changing Policies and Procedures

I just had to name the chapter after the main source of the problem. The initialism PDPM in a SNF is just about equivalent to that point in a movie when the helpless damsel runs into a corner with no escape, and her killer is staring her right in the eyes.

# P.D.P.M.

# AHHHHHH!!!

### RUG IV TO PDPM

Once upon a time, patients who came to a nursing facility to rehabilitate from their illnesses were

classified under:[1]

- Rehabilitation plus Extensive Services.
- Ultra High Rehabilitation.
- Very High Rehabilitation.
- High Rehabilitation.
- Medium Rehabilitation.
- Low Rehabilitation.
- Extensive Services.
- Special Care High.

- Special Care Low.
- Clinically Complex.

Now, each service has a category:

- Nursing.
- ST.
- PT.
- OT.

Furthermore, each patient has a classifier under each category. Those that apply to us SLPs are SA, SB, SC, SD, SE, SF, SG, SH, SI, SJ, SK, and SL.

Until October 1, 2019, facilities received payments through Medicare Part A insurance as the patient stayed. Now, the payment model provides an allowance under the prospective payment system (PPS). This payment to the facility is determined by assessments completed in the minimum data set (MDS), which will document various areas of the patient's overall function. How complete the patient's history and report are determine the score (or points). The more information the facility has, the better they can justify a score. More points mean more money. The patient will likely receive rehab services, but especially so if they are not considered 'skilled' by nursing. This means their diagnoses do not require a high level of care to manage, or that their overall independence in obtaining their daily needs is high. A patient that is skilled by nursing may have wounds, not be able to walk, have tube feedings, require respiratory assistance, or have an otherwise unstable health status.

Under the previously used RUG-IV system, these assessments were done on days 5, 14, 30, 60, and 90. According to the fact sheet provided by the Center for Medicare and Medicaid Services, an unscheduled assessment could occur when the patient experienced a significant change or an increase or decrease in therapy volume. On the Patient Driven Payment Model (PDPM) schedule, these assessment reference dates (ARD) were changed to one look-back period of days 1-8, which would then cover the rest of the patient's stay up to 100 days of Medicare Part A, given there was no significant change or discharge from the facility, which would require an interim payment assessment (IPA) or PPS discharge, respectively.

## Initial MDS Screening

The sections of the MDS that refer to us SLPs are Sections C (cognitive patterns) and K (swallowing and nutritional status). Naturally, I was accustomed to never really having to hear about the MDS much; social work handled our sections for cognitive patterns, and the dietician handled our sections for swallowing and nutritional status. In the months leading up to the implementation of the new model, I was unpleasantly introduced to a number of new forms that I had to assess each Med A patient on. One was the BIMS—the Brief Interview of Mental Status. Despite its drawbacks, it gives a score based on short-term memory and orientation to time, a two-minute assessment at most for some key information. Then, there was another form that would determine a score for the Speech component on the MDS. While not very lengthy, this one is a little more complicated, so let me break it down a bit.

The sections include:[2]

NEUROLOGIC DISORDER versus NON-NEUROLOGIC DISORDER.

While a neurologic disorder generally refers to a patient that is post-stroke, non-neurologic indicates that the PDPM clinical category will be in major joint replacement, orthopedic surgery, non-orthopedic surgery, acute infection, cardiovascular and coagulations, pulmonary, non-surgical orthopedic/musculoskeletal, cancer, or medical management. You will not be required to specify which of these categories it is, just that it is non-neurologic.

CONCURRENT DISABILITY OR SLP COMORBIDITY

This includes Aphasia, Laryngeal Cancer, CVA,TIA, or Stroke, Apraxia, Hemiplegia or Hemiparesis, Dysphagia (following stroke),Traumatic Brain Injury, ALS, Tracheostomy (while Resident), Oral Cancers, Ventilator (while Resident), or Speech & Language Deficits.

COGNITIVE IMPAIRMENT refers to:

- Cognitively Intact 13–15, of which the CPS Score is 0.
- Mildly Impaired 8–12, of which the CPS Score is 1–2.
- Moderately Impaired 0–7, of which the CPS Score is 3–4.
- Severely Impaired –99, of which the CPS Score is 5–6.

When the patient is unable to complete or participate in the assessment, we score 99.

SWALLOWING DISORDER refers to the:

- Loss of liquids/solids from the mouth during eating/drinking.
- Holding food in the mouth/cheeks or residual food in the mouth after meals.
- Coughing or choking during meals or when swallowing medications.
- Complaints of difficulty or pain with swallowing.

ALTERED DIET

This refers to whether the patient has an altered food or liquid consistency. Note that the patient will not apply for this reimbursement section if they are on a tube-feeding program.

# CLUTCHING MY PEARLS... THERAPY ON A SATURDAY!?

They officially established PDPM on October 1, 2019. We spent months and months in training and meetings to discuss everything that would change, and when that change finally occurred, it was a surprise that every nursing home didn't burst right into flames.

My facility went from having five to six days of physical and occupational therapy to seven, then to strictly five. Speech generally only had five days, but advanced to six to seven days right along with the other rehab services, requiring an SLP to cover a weekend day.

Me? Working on Saturdays?

What kind of dark world were they creating for us? Not too long after, it was thankfully limited to five days only for rehab therapy, so my glorified Monday-through-Friday schedule was restored. (Note: this is 'as needed', and other rehab facilities have maintained six to seven days to satisfy patients who prefer to be seen ASAP, or just to evade weekend-long periods of inactivity.)

Most changes corrected after several weeks or months into using the new model:

- In our facility, the initial cognitive screens (BIMS) for the MDS have returned to the care of the social worker, but we still take the burden of Section K for paper only, meaning someone else is responsible for entering it onto the MDS system.
- Two-week courses of therapy were encouraged, almost mandated, for a long-term patient. Towards the end of my time at the SNF, I was hardly ever bothered about a therapy course that lasted less than a month. In reality, CMS wants to see therapy courses with more minutes or a similar amount to the previous year. A decrease in therapy minutes raises red flags; however, it is more difficult under this system to maintain long therapy courses when the patient benefits from all three rehab services.
- My facility encouraged me to treat concurrently and in groups as often as possible at the start, but later this was not a mandate. Therefore, group therapy was rarely a part of my daily activities.

Needless to say, your facility might do this all the way different. It seemed like the introduction of PDPM had everyone on their toes, until it happened and we weren't doing everything wrong after all, out of the way of having to bill and screen a little differently. Without any transition period, and no room for mistakes, it's understandable. What remains, and may still affect you as an SLP in this setting, is that:

- ST and PT share the same $2,000 allowance from Medicare for Part B patients—OT gets their own $2,000 allowance. However, the cap is transparent and a higher allowance may be reviewed for services exceeding the threshold.
- ST will need a measurable growth outcome that can be achieved in less time.
- SLP and other rehab presence will be virtually minimized as needed. Even with a growing number of patients, these times call for specified amounts of providers to work within the facility. Coverages for caseloads that are too heavy are a thing of the past. In my

facility, holding therapy became the new etiquette.

- Communication and training will be even more necessary.
- Screening and attention to long-term care (LTC) patients will be critical to maintaining a caseload.
- Diversification of skills to identify viable areas of interest for rehabilitation will be appreciated.

With PDPM, we were over-prepared. This is only a portion of the endless changes you can experience as you work in a SNF. In other cases, you might step left and right to avoid running over toes over a change you didn't even know was happening. Generally, we take orders from the state, and it is needless to say that they never make up their minds. This was most evident in the crisis occurring after the end of February 2020. We'll get to that, but for now, the survival tactic for this chapter is to foresee the unforeseen, ask plenty of questions, and prepare yourself daily for something unexpected, so as to not catch yourself on the wrong side of a new procedure. Also, beware of the in-service, in-service, in-service approach, to the point of nails digging into your skin on information we all already know: dementia indicators, safety, fire procedures. Then, for once, when it matters that we all know what's going on, we hear about it through the grapevine!

**CHAPTER FOOTNOTES**

[1]https://www.cms.gov/Medicare/Medicare-Fee-for-Service-Payment/SNFPPS/Downloads/PDPM_Fact_Sheet_AdminPresumption_v6_508.pdf

[2]https://www.cms.gov/Medicare/Medicare-Fee-for-Service-Payment/SNFPPS/Downloads/MLN_CalL_PDPM_Presentation_508.pdf

# Part Four
# LONG-TERM PATIENT CARE

# 14

# THE PEOPLE ARE SEEING GHOSTS

*A Guide to Thriving with Dementia*

Every SNF is unique, but, for sure, every facility has a percentage of patients who present with dementia. In some, there are whole units dedicated to caring for patients with severe cases of behavioral issues. There's no way to prepare you adequately for what you may encounter. I'd say this group of people is the least predictable. With this diagnosis, we have to expect the unexpected and creatively move around each obstacle. Here are some stories.

## STORY TIME WITH GUY
### Impulse Wins the Race

Guy was a very confused man with an unsteady gait. He loved to walk miles and miles around the unit with me on his arm as often as possible. If I encouraged him to sit so we could work on our sessions, he'd pull me from my seat aggressively. Sometimes, walking and talking and finding a calm moment to take a sip of juice or a sandwich bite was the best we could do. When it came to the food and drink trials, he needed to be watched like a hawk. If you let him hold any food by himself, he'd fit it into his mouth whole. With liquids, he gulped and gulped and gulped almost until he could have possibly drowned in the juice.

**WHAT WORKED**

Self-control and awareness was out the window, but providing hand-over-hand and consistent reinforcement reduced Guy's tendency to grab and gulp down food. I did not expect a patient like this to come to a point of independence; however, even if we can reduce the help needed just a little, we call it a win.

## STORY TIME WITH GLORIA
### Pump the Brakes

When I had met Gloria, she could walk and eat by herself. She declined fairly quickly to a point of sitting in a recliner chair, sleeping away about 90% of the day, and being completely fruitless in her daily activities. Her dysphagia problem quickly grew to a severe level and before long, she was on PEG tube feeding for failure to thrive. During our sessions, she screamed at the top of her lungs every time someone touched her. She usually refused to open her mouth for trials, and spat out liquids whenever she accepted them.

## WHAT WORKED

We did mostly sensory activities, which worked to some extent to reduce her negative reaction to things touching or nearing her mouth. Instead of a spoon, I used a toothette dipped in thickened juice. The screaming subsided during trials, and she eventually accepted a full spoon. Like the stock market, therapy is never consistently upwards, though we wish to cash out on every progress note. In the end, Gloria unfortunately could not achieve a pleasure diet, but the work we did that advanced her abilities even just a little may have created the hope for a future opportunity to work together again. This I consider a win, as well.

In cases like this one, I'll make a point that if it's difficult to justify that feeding is a 'pleasurable' activity, it's perfectly okay to back out. Sometimes, this is not a total loss. Dementia patients can exhibit spontaneous changes in both directions, though we typically attend to the declining aspect of things.

# STORY TIME WITH COLETTE
## *Take Me Back to Florida*

Colette's family was adamant about beginning cognitive-communication therapy to help improve her orientation and memory. She was having trouble adjusting after moving from a different state. She thought she was visiting with her daughter in her house and didn't recall that her husband had passed. For her, everything was temporary, although she was really there for long-term care. In the following months, she declined significantly. She hardly spoke and stared into space when anyone called her name. Then she developed difficulties with feeding as well, including trouble chewing and holding food in her mouth. At times, she couldn't even trigger a swallow.

## WHAT WORKED

Communication strategies worked significantly better than any traditional swallow exercises I would usually do with a patient. Although she wasn't as verbal as at first, she could respond to most yes or no questions, which allowed me to guide and assist in the process of feeding her. Because she became emotional during our sessions,

I thought of creating a communication board for her to express her feelings in the moment. In being able to identify the pictures, I knew that she was aware of being tired or sad. Her responses to feeding were directly related to those feelings. Her frustration was reduced by allowing her to exercise some repetitive but non-dangerous behaviors, by attending to her emotions, and allowing rest when she needed it.

# STORY TIME WITH DONNA
## I Hate You, but not on Sundays

In Intent (chapter 4), I mentioned that NYC is my melting pot. Donna, whom I had on my caseload on several occasions, is an example of why that part is so important to me. This patient was about 95 years old-a sweet talker, decorated with Catholic inspired jewelry and inspirational quotes on the walls of her room, and loved to get her hair colored and curled on Tuesdays. Actually, she was quite a predictable woman amongst most with her kind of diagnosis. The therapy process, however, didn't turn out nearly as expected. In the first place, she suffered a stroke in the middle of her rehab therapy with the PT, and when she returned from the hospital, she had right-sided hemiplegia, a facial droop, and a severe dysphagia problem. As expected, I put her on my caseload, and while she made some progress, it was with a lot of patience and encouragement. She hated oral motor and pharyngeal exercises, and getting her to participate was difficult since she wasn't aware of her problem even after frequent and thorough explanations of it.

Long story short, this patient came to hate me-like, really hate me. At least her dementia convinced her that I was a terrible person. She threw down anything I put in front of her and even hit me once when I sat next to her. She called me names and used racial slurs. Once, later on, I thought that she might have forgotten everything that we'd been through. I didn't, but I was pressured constantly to try again with her. This time, she participated for the duration of the evaluation. A success! I thought. On day two, she wouldn't allow me to come within three feet of her. She had hands swinging if I even tried it. Guys, I was asking staff to give her food trials so that I could observe her from the corner of the room or from behind a curtain, and even that wasn't successful when she could guess the cookie came from me.

## WHAT WORKED

With this patient, honestly, almost nothing worked. I did what I could, in the way of fighting for an objective test, providing education upon more education, and using the other humans around me to draw results. What I can say is that changing my mindset worked. I didn't take the things she did or said personally. Instead, I took the time and patience I could muster to remain respectful and think of new ideas; I communicated with other professionals and her family about our experience. When all was said and done, I avoided working with her—as far as reasonably possible.

# CAN'T BELIEVE IT'S NOT DEMENTIA!
*Being Mindful of Dementia-like Disorders*

While "dementia" is becoming quite the ubiquitous diagnosis—sources report that diagnostic assessments for Alzheimer's disease specifically have high sensitivity with relatively low specificity, meaning that there is a premise for over-diagnosis—you may come across presentations of dementia-like symptoms that don't come with any cognitive or neuropathic diagnoses. In some cases, these symptoms lend themselves to another illness being treated[1].

Heart, liver, and kidney disease are famous for their perfect pairing with reduced cognitive function. As these chronic illnesses progress, it often affects a patient's attention, memory, safety awareness, and response time.

Depression and anxiety are often overlooked as indicators or risk factors for cognitive issues and dementia-like symptoms in the SNF setting. However, it is certain that these fast-developing conditions mirror social withdrawal and the deficits of concentration, memory, and judgement.

Neuropathic diagnoses such as traumatic brain injuries or idiopathic normal pressure hydrocephalus are examples of diagnoses that can present with concomitant progressive cognitive deficits, similar to dementia[2]. In fact, it is not odd to find that a patient has a dual diagnosis. While it is important to know the difference so you can treat with a plan in mind, I find that the treatment does not differ significantly. In the end, we don't know what is going to become of the patient. We don't know that the illness will improve or that cognition will be restored fully, even in the case of a virtually complete recovery. When the person returns to the community, or begins a new life in our little long-term care community, it's our job to ensure that they have the tools they need to reach the highest possible quality of living.

Most of these don't seem like true thriving, but while you are just a human fighting a disease of God, the devil, mother nature, or what have you, your tug in the right direction is meaningful and appreciated. Your dementia survival guide is just to maintain your patience and stick to the plan, but expect nothing. I've beat myself up over situations like these in the past, and thought of everything I could have done beyond everything I had already done to make my plan work. In this case, dementia is no one's decision, but it is everyone's reality. The more everyone can band together, the better the outcome for the patient.

**CHAPTER FOOTNOTES**

[1]Beach, Thomas G., Sarah E. Monsell, Leslie E. Phillips, and Walter Kukull. "Accuracy of the Clinical Diagnosis of Alzheimer Disease at National Institute on Aging Alzheimer Disease Centers, 2005–2010." Oxford AcademicJournal of Neuropathology & Experimental Neurology. Journal of Neuropathology & Experimental Neurology, Volume 71, Issue 4, April 2012, Pages 266–273, April 1, 2012. https://academic.oup.com/jnen/article/71/4/266/2917384.

[2]"2020 Alzheimer's Disease Facts and Figures." Alzheimers & Dementia: The Journal of the Alzheimer's Association 16: 391–460., March 10, 2020. https://alz-journals.onlinelibrary.wiley.com/doi/full/10.1002/alz.12068.

# 15

# WE'VE COME THIS FAR BY FAITH

*A Guide to Caring for the Declining or Stagnant Patient*

A long-term setting is easily described as the gray area of nursing and medical facilities. While never quite completely dying down on the 'action,' it's certainly not your local emergency room. It's a purgatory between home and hell. You will remember these words and understand why I said it once you've come to know the setting well enough.

Even if the premise is initially short-term rehab, it often becomes long-term or somewhere in the middle—maybe several months. This happens when the patient is not progressing fast enough or to a satisfactory level. Families are placed in the tough position of turning over the responsibility of Mom-Mom and Pop-Pop's immediate care to complete strangers. Managing this transition into a new way of living is especially difficult for the patient, who may experience cycles of emotional vulnerability or even show unusual behaviors.

Where the emotional transition is only a piece of the puzzle, the prognosis of the patient's disease remains a strong factor in the family's decisions, in coordination with the healthcare staff such as the social worker, doctor, and nurse. If a full recovery is not foreseen, management is the next best option. When the prognosis is poor, it is likely to result in a significant loss of independence, quality of life, or possibly even death.

At any level, we are intimately involved as it is fit for the patient. What is within our skill set may not be an immediate need for the patient. However, for one that is declining, it is suspected that health issues related to the heart, lungs, kidneys, and neurological function will require our intervention for swallowing, voice, and cognitive-communication.

To manage and leverage our intervention in these patients' lives, there are a few terminologies that we should get familiar with. Not all of them directly apply to us, but we'll come across them often and they help us to better understand the kind of patients we're dealing with.

## PALLIATIVE CARE

You've likely heard this term at least once if you have been pursuing the medical setting for some time. Palliative care is a wide and general term for what we do, usually with more elderly patients or those more advanced in disease. The use of the term 'palliative care' considers that the patient is terminally ill. One does not, however, need to be close to death in order to receive this sort of care. Examples of frequented diseases or illnesses that we come across that warrant palliative care include heart disease, lung disease, cancer, multiple sclerosis, kidney disease, and dementia. Palliative care is a holistic approach that considers the spiritual and emotional needs of the patient just as much as his or her physical and medical needs. The information in the advance directive may guide our access to a patient during palliative care. I'll explain its components below.

## ADVANCED DIRECTIVES

### Full Code

'Full code' only refers to the patient's desire for cardiopulmonary resuscitation (CPR) or electrical shock to the heart in the event that the patient is not breathing or shows no pulse. This code status, outlined in the advance directive, essentially means the patient is saying, "No matter what, I want to live." While I'd always believed this code status indicated an underlying stability of health, I've come to realize it is an extremely personal decision. Though there are long-term patients with full code orders who fall considerably lower on the bill of health, more often than not, we consider a semi-independent and alert patient with few concerns for an exacerbation of internal chemistry. When that profile is not so, especially when you know a patient hasn't been doing too well for a while, it's usually at this time that the patient's family is overdue for a meeting to discuss a plan for an extreme event. Where our service is concerned, we are allowed any method of intervention that falls within our scope of practice, including dysphagia assessment, treatment, referral for objective studies, and justification for PEG tube placement.

### DNR/DNI

A patient's advance directive may specify DNR (do not resuscitate) only or DNR and DNI (do not intubate). Respectively, these medical abbreviations indicate that a patient is not to receive life-saving measures to restart the heart through cardiopulmonary resuscitation (CPR) or to restore breathing through respiratory intubation. Another abbreviation sometimes paired to these is ADN (allow natural death). A family may decide on this directive because it's likely that the person receiving the treatment views the heroic act as 'unnatural' or extensive. It is also possible that if the life-saving procedure is successful, the revived patient's loved ones may view them as a completely different person, because they may behave differently. For example, Sweet Aunt Karen, who was very talkative and had a great appetite, was resuscitated and became Aunt Karen, who couldn't lift her head or her hand to feed herself. With reduced responsiveness to medication, we knew Aunt Karen's heart problems were worsening and realized that eventually her heart would possibly fail. For the duration of Karen's stay in the SNF, we want to ensure the least amount of suffering and the greatest quality of life in her waning hours, days, or months. Within our scope, all treatments are allowed, but it is important to consider how extensive interventions (e.g., a PEG tube) may affect the care of patients like Karen and their families, who may be averse to such treatments. In addition to DNR/DNI, a patient's advance directive may also indicate that they must be put on comfort care.

## Comfort Care

In a long-term setting, 'comfort care' is a term you will definitely come across. This is an agreement between the healthcare staff and family, which is signed as a legal document on the Medical Orders for Life-Sustaining Treatment (MOLST). By this point, the patient has exhausted several options to treat a disease or disorder, and has had to realize that it wasn't getting better. For quality of life to be preserved, families ensure that these patients are not extensively treated. This is not the same as the patient's DNR/DNI status, but is typically paired with it, and sometimes the refusal of hospitalization, too. Life-sustaining treatments, such as a PEG tube, are also typically refused as a part of this agreement. There is still a little wiggle room with comfort care, though much of a SLP's intervention is limited. We aren't likely to see a full restoration of function, and should not expect so. In this case, we want to keep the therapy short and sweet and focused on comfort, compensatory strategies, and caregiver training above anything else. Again, it is crucial to consider and communicate with the family to understand what they are comfortable with, regarding the provision of care for their loved one. It is key to have a good grasp on the patient's case and to share educational material on the usefulness of the procedure to illustrate how it could impact on their quality of life.

## Hospice

'Hospice' usually means an immediate cessation of all treatments related to the patient's primary and most progressive disease, cessation of rehab therapy, and that the patient is most probably in a bed-bound status. Patients are assumed to be 'ready to die' and only necessary procedures, such as cleaning, changing, and feeding are to continue. In some cases, patients may still receive medication for symptoms not related to their primary diagnosis, or to reduce their pain. Where feeding is concerned, the speech pathologist may be allowed to see a patient for an evaluation-only or continued treatment with the permission of hospice coordinators, doctor, and family. Hospice treatment is atypical and should only be held out as long as is absolutely necessary for the patient to achieve an adequate level of safety. This may be day-to-day testing and observation or training of the nursing staff. The purpose is never the patient's improvement, as the hospice status indicates that the patient is not likely to improve, and it would be unethical to impose those measures.

The graveness of some of these topics may initially bring heartbreak, but one thing to realize is that the patient is being protected and served in a way that preserves their dignity and freedom to live and die as naturally as possible. In no case is the patient sure to wither immediately, nor are there any promises of a long life to come. Given the facts of the disease with which the patient has been diagnosed, physicians can decide if 'life as usual' is an option. Almost always in the long-term setting, it's not. When they notice a severe decline, nursing staff need to be prepared to react appropriately to it. The information that we find within the chart about these recommendations are necessary to us SLPs as well, to help us serve the patient as ethically and usefully as possible.

Despite typically riding along the plateau, the long-term patient can pique the least bit of hope for improvements, no matter their code status. Some—though not many—families choose to keep a full code status for a patient all the way into hospice care. These situations have less to do with rules; rather, it is more about considerations and the values of the patient and family you are working with. It is mainly important to know what these statuses are and what they mean for your patient, so you know how to proceed properly with your intervention.

Regular screening gives us the opportunity to identify cases that may have fallen completely off of the radar. In many cases, patients have a greater ability to succeed in therapy the second or third time around than upon their initial admission to the facility. It can be redundant to go through sheets and sheets of people who have SLP-related comorbidities with no true positive projection, nor any changes. When you do find a diamond in the rough, it can have amazing outcomes.

## STORY TIME WITH DOC
### PEG Tube Weaning

My first complete PEG tube wean was with a man, whom we will call Doc. Doc was post-stroke, with limited verbalizations, and severe contractures that limited his ability to maintain correct positioning for feeding. He did not have the profile of a very strong candidate, but given that he was able to trigger a swallow and was susceptible to passive techniques, I took a shot and we went for the long-haul. It took months to see the full weaning process through. Getting an objective test scheduled takes weeks to forever for a long-term care professional. I actually had to discharge Doc from therapy after making significant gains, just to wait for the MBS results to come back. (Not every facility will want you to do this, so check with your department leaders and your supervisor.) Anyway, after that delay we were onward and upward. He achieved pleasure feeding, followed by successive meals, and finally a full oral diet, which meant no more PEG tube feeding. After a year of not eating anything, it was a huge hurdle to overcome. This was over one year ago, and I saw him again recently to continue the progress that we once made prior to a plateau.

The nursing staff can be helpful in identifying residents who are ready for a change of some sort. In fact, some will be so helpful as to get a jump start on your therapy for you. Mind the sarcasm—this is not okay, but it happens.

## STORY TIME WITH PENELOPE
### Miracles Do Happen

Once, I found a nursing staff feeding bread to a patient on a strictly puree diet with no allowances. This patient happened to be on honey-thick liquids, and for God knows how long, she was naturally improving without ever being seen for therapy. This makes clear the usefulness of screening, which I suppose, for some reason, she never received. My reaction was to pick up immediately and gently in-service the staff on precautions and the referral process. Upon evaluation, I found that Penelope ate and drank like a well-developed teenager. No problems in sight. During her short course of therapy, she presented with minimal concerns for mastication, but I struggled to find even a hair of deficit in anything else. I asked myself how does someone magically recover to this extent without being noticed? It turned out that I would find this sort of situation plenty more times, though not as extreme.

In other cases, you won't be so lucky to behold a magic trick of nature or to pull all the way through notable gains and change lives for the better. Sometimes, the therapy turns out to make do. By that, I mean you learn what your patient responds to, what they like, and what their family's perspective is. With all that, you seek to make the situation manageable rather than to improve it. It's at times like these you have to communicate at your optimal potential, because everyone's eyes are on you to make the decisions that matter.

# STORY TIME WITH TAKI
## *Finger Foods*

Taki was a sweet old lady with a mean sting during meal times. Taki did not usually like to have people feed her, but she was also pretty bad at doing it herself. She was great at holding her own cup but couldn't, for goodness' sake, place food onto a spoon. She liked to use her hands to eat, but since she'd declined in function in the previous months, she could no longer eat the items she used to. As a result, she'd been downgraded to puree, which was a big deal for her family.

On her second round of therapy, I attempted to trial chopped solids, hoping to upgrade her diet, eventually. In the meantime, I worked on increasing her intake of puree meals and verbally educating the nursing staff about her need for strong encouragement and assistance. Being that she had poor oral reception to spoons, I had to work under some fierce circumstances. I felt a bit like a mad scientist, finding ways to make food stick to the convex portion of a spoon or to not fall out of the concave portion when it was upside down. Then, I went to the length of using a second spoon to scoop the food out of the original spoon into the oral cavity. Creativity is key, but is often lost in the carryover.

During our sessions, she ate 80% of her meals, but 5% at best with the nursing staff. Unfortunately, everyone became frustrated. Me, because I continued to find her sitting alone with food in front of her on a table, unable to do anything with it except place her fingers in it and have things fall over. The CNAs, because I kept asking them why no one was assisting her. The nursing supervisor, because I kept reminding her to enforce the recommendation and ensure the staff were involved. The patient's daughter, because not only did she prefer her mother to be on a chopped solid diet; she also brought food for her every Wednesday, just to find out her mother had already eaten. The social worker, because she got a great deal of the backlash. Above all, the patient-because all these people were standing around her geri chair, screaming at each other while it was already 1 PM, and she hadn't eaten since breakfast!

This is the kind of case that results in the decision that never appears, at surface level, to be the most perfectly outlined plan or solution. It's just what has to work. Because Taki was not a strong aspiration risk, it was feasible to justify an upgrade to chopped solids based on the family's wishes and the patient's more frequent acceptance. I made it a point that the patient's family was educated about the risks, but they insisted. As the patient was on comfort care, not one complaint was ever whispered about the situation again, and the patient lived what seemed to be 'happily ever after' until her time came to pass away peacefully.

You sometimes run into the situation that once you make a recommendation and communicate it to the staff, everyone is too afraid or too impatient to carry it out. Other times, the effort is overzealous and valiant to overstep the recommendations and do what one sees fit. Families will, predictably, take the latter route.

## STORY TIME WITH SANTANA
### Family Has the Last Say

Santana was peacefully hanging out in her geri chair or in bed from day to day for at least over a year since I'd known her. With dementia, it's unpredicted exactly what time and on what day one will spark a significant change in behavior or function. Santana got very sick and was hospitalized for a week or two. When she came back, she had no diet recommendations, whatsoever. This is extremely unusual, since she also didn't have an alternative means of consuming daily nutrition. According to the SLP at the hospital, she couldn't complete an evaluation, because Santana simply refused everything they offered her. Thankfully, when I saw her, she was willing to accept the trials; unfortunately, she did poorly with all oral trials. I seconded the previous health professionals' recommendations for a PEG tube. The family was in strong disagreement. They fought this until the very end. It was a blessing that Santana started to tolerate more food for a short time, but it was almost a rush to get a diet set in place that she didn't really seem ready for. She was weak at times and couldn't finish her meals. The story ends the way it ends, and it isn't for the better or the worse, really.

It didn't matter whether or not I sided with the family in this case. I didn't have to. While I could spend my energy focusing on my recommendations and convincing families to exchange their ideas for mine, I think it's an unethical way to carry out an intervention. You'll find that some SLPs are like this, and it's usually because they care so much. For me, however, it is just this kind of freedom that comes along with a patient living for comfort and not to regain their youth or prolong unnecessary suffering.

This is why people have proxies and those that know them well, so that you don't have to press on what would be best for them after the five to fifteen minutes you were present at the bedside. Not to say that it isn't enough time to get a grasp, but it sure isn't enough to make a life-changing decision. That's why those decisions were made before the patient's decline, before you arrived at their bedside, and before there was any platform on which to disagree.

## A GUIDE TO THE CARE PLAN MEETING

At my facility, I was rarely invited to attend care plan meetings, even if the patient was diagnosed with dysphagia and was carrying out a plan to achieve gains in that area. The times I was present were when the family was especially concerned about feeding and wanted to hear from me directly. The best way to go about discussing your patient's case during a care plan meeting is to:

- Provide all background history that you are aware of.
- Note what you've observed while working with the patient.
- Discuss what has been successful and unsuccessful.
- Allow the family to give feedback.
- Provide recommendations that are considerate of the family's wishes.
- Provide a reasonable prognosis, expectations, and dates to follow up.

This chapter is entitled We've Come This Far By Faith because beyond everything we've learned in school and on the job, and beyond whatever the patient, family, and physician have decided and outlined in the advance directive, lies the faith that it will be enough. That's all we have. We can't change minds or perform miracles, but we can continue to educate ourselves and others involved in the patient's care to do our best to obtain the best outcome possible.

# 16

# MOM AND POP

## A Guide to Managing Death and Dying

No matter what changes procedurally in the facility, in a long-term care setting, you have the joy of caring for the same patients over and again. It's one thing that never tired me about being in this sort of setting. I quite strongly dislike repetition in most cases, but it's pleasurable that I could build a rapport that lasted for a long time, which allowed me to follow and notice changes in people I treated over time. Some bonds are built over days, and some over—well—two years. Some will begin to feel closer to you as you get to know them and their families. The way you value your patient's happiness and quality of life will be evident to those you see in a long-term setting. You may have joked with them, cried with them, or been their confidante. You never forget that their time is limited, and that alone may break you when you know their time is near.

# STORY TIME WITH EDDIE
## Nakuombea Maisha Marefu

The most significant loss for me was a friend of mine, Eddie. Eddie's stay at the facility was fairly short, compared to most. He was a long-time smoker who had a diagnosis of pulmonary fibrosis—a disease in which scar tissues form inside the lungs and restricts breathing. This progressed to a fatal level in a matter of months. The prognosis was poor from his admission, but it was still such a surprising and soul-binding turn when he began to look and feel like someone who was passing.

He was someone who believed strongly in God and religion, and he shared his convictions with me as often as he could. As much as he was the one going through suffering, he always found time to ask me how I was doing. He asked for favor after favor, which I didn't mind at all; however, in aspects that related to my job, I felt useless, because his condition caused him to be uncomfortable no matter what measures anyone took. The ideals of the rehab team are to create a system that allows the patient to manage activities of daily living as best as possible to retain the highest possible quality of life. I couldn't give that to him. As much as he hated the food he received, he couldn't manage swallowing anything but puree. The mucus that held his throat hostage constantly made him feel like he was unable to get a free and clear breath, especially when eating. He lost weight at an intense rate. When he was given a PEG tube to manage it, it made him nauseous, and eventually he became too sick to receive feeding.

Eddie could not win this battle. I didn't cry when he passed, because I had grieved on so many other occasions when he was in need and begging to die. When the day finally came, I felt a sense of relief for him, with an accompanied weight of sadness for his family, who would have done anything to hold on to him for a little while longer.

The Swahili phrase 'nakuombea maisha marefu' means: "I pray for you a long life."

Eddie wasn't the first nor the last, but with each patient that goes and each family that suffers, we hold a very special responsibility to be communicative, patient, and kind. It is not the time for reprimanding a family or a patient, which we may be inclined to do when they're bringing the wrong foods and not following through with the strategies we taught. Instead, it's the time to remind them that they are doing their best, and their Mom-Mom and Pop-Pop really need them at that moment. Families are so much more receptive to our professional and calm behavior when they realize their family member is becoming more and more fragile.

We should take advantage of the unknown length of time we have to serve our patients, to bring opportunities to the table which everyone else has forgotten about. We don't get enough credit for how prominent our role is at the end-of-life care of patients when other rehab therapies have long let go. Delusions and dementia are not exclusionary criteria for having someone to listen. Old age is not an indicator of a lesser desire for independence of thought and action. In their later years, no one wants to be made out as a child, despite the famous saying. Yet, it seems a regular occurrence that these people are scolded and told what they can't have.

It's our responsibility to hear them out.

Sometimes death is expected, slow, and solemn. Other times, it is unexpected, sudden, and extremely unsettling. I can't say that when you start therapy with a patient, you'll know it's something you will have to be a part of, unless you are managing a hospice patient, in which case the beginning and end of your intervention is quite clearly defined.

## THE LAST WORDS...

No case is the same, but there are a few key signals and events leading up to this point you should be aware of that might happen, and that you will need to remain abreast of:

### Feeding Issues/Dysphagia

- Whether you have made gains or have been stagnant throughout the course of therapy thus far, someone who is dying may present new problems with feeding, or an exacerbation of an existing dysphagia.
- When the problem has exacerbated beyond the patient's ability to tolerate any intake, the doctor may make an order for NPO, or for the patient not to be fed. If there is a PEG tube in place, this will become the primary source of nutrition. If not, the patient will be left to rest peacefully without being introduced to food during the day. If the patient is on hospice care, no alternative means of nutrition will be put in place.
- When the patient is placed on hospice care, dysphagia therapy should immediately cease. In special cases, the hospice may reimburse for end-of-life SLP care, but justification for this rehab service is key, which I discussed in We've Come This Far By Faith. If hospice care is not considered, dysphagia therapy should end if the patient does not show any improvement over several days.
- Dysphagia therapy continues if there is no NPO order and the patient is not completely safe on even the most restrictive diet. Additional diet modifications and training for caregivers and nursing staff about positioning and precautions should take place. In case all else fails, you should discuss a possible order for NPO or alternative nutrition (by IV fluid) with the physician. A new PEG tube is not a reasonable consideration for someone who appears to be dying as a result of medical conditions unrelated to nutrition.

## Lethargy / Minimal Participation

- A patient who is very lethargic may still benefit from passive techniques and stimulation to complete oral and pharyngeal exercise. This might help to increase their tolerance and endurance for meals, but should not be extensive or intended to advance the diet consistency. It is intended to manage the problem, and should be discontinued if the patient seems uncomfortable.
- A patient that is unable to participate in your intervention should not remain on your caseload for an extended period. Start training the caregivers as soon as possible and look to the rehab director for insight about a discharge date.

## Confusion

A person who is dying might likely be confused or unreasonable. Remain patient and anticipate their needs as much as possible and always document any communication with other staff.

## Asking for Water Frequently/Peculiar Food Desires

- Our role in this situation is extremely complicated. Knowing that someone who is sick, and not expected to get any better, has one dying wish, you want to help them get it. Patients who are NPO unfortunately will not be granted water or any other request for PO.
- Patients with thickened liquids may have trouble tolerating the water, and for those who don't like the thickened water, it really presents a loss for them. Flexibility can be given when the patient's caregivers are aware of how to administer an allowed volume or type of desired item or liquid, and the potential risks that are associated with doing so. Consider a protocol similar to that of free water, or try carbonated or sparkling water as an alternative.

## Frequently with Family

- The best thing you can do for a family during this time is to respect their time and privacy with their loved one. You may have to readjust your schedule several times to allow for this. Take some time to inform them of precautions and updates, and encourage them— they will also be noticeably unwell.

## Unusual Behaviors

- Be sure to report and document non-functional and unsafe behaviors (these may be sexual in nature or lead to frequent falls).
- Be non-judgmental and support your patient as well as you can.
- Redirect the patient towards functional behaviors.

## Unusual Requests

- Some of your dying patients will yearn for the moment they can be relieved of their discomfort and pain. Patients have asked me to help them approach the finish line. Obviously, this is not within any scope of my practice or beliefs, and it was difficult to stay ahead when this happened during each session. It is important to stay calm, not make any promises that can't be fulfilled, and consult mental health or chaplain services when it's appropriate. You will also be in the position to provide coping and counseling strategies to carry on.

When all is said and done, death and dying takes a toll on you—the therapist—to some degree. You may feel affected by the passing of someone you treated, and the process of dying can last hours, or it can last months. It is not fair to have to be a part of this process and to never be a part of the grief. It's not unusual or out of place to seek your own strategies for coping or mental health intervention to manage being in this sort of environment.

# 17

# NAKED PEOPLE

## *A Guide to Managing Patients' Privacy*

Naked is both a literal and metaphorical reference here. Naturally, when in someone's home, you will become the beneficiary of learning deeply personal things about their lifestyle. Stay for a while, and you'll get to notice pictures on the wall of a family reunion or a trinket from their home country. A while longer, and you'll learn that they snore when they sleep and have a bad habit of biting their nails. See them for swallow therapy, and you'll be all too aware of the shapes and colors of the insides of their mouth, plus that one spot that they can't reach with their tongue. You'll know that if you see them anywhere between 10 AM–12 PM, you'll have to center their speech-language activity around Let's Make a Deal or The Price is Right, because they won't miss either for the world. You'll know the things they're likely to remember, and won't be surprised about the things they forget. You'll find yourself pouring coffee or tea—you'll know their preference—to an exact point of a cup, knowing that it's the right amount they will need to clear each bite of a slice of bread and butter.

I say all this to say: in a setting like this, you'll get to know most of your patients just about as well as an extended family member. Likely even better. Our patients bare more and more of themselves to us the longer they stay and the longer we stick around. It's why the workplace becomes so much more than just your job. It's why we're keen on seeing changes and equipped to respond to them. It's also why, when they go, it takes a little piece of us with them.

Given that you have all of this information, it becomes key to the way you manage their treatment, and you also have an upper hand in training others on how to care for them. Between staff, you discuss patients in passing quite often, usually to ask questions related to how they're eating, how they're participating in another therapy, how to motivate or make them happy, and what some of their preferences are. These passing conversations, in my opinion, turn out to be the best way of managing the patient, because everyone comes closer to being on the same page even though they can't all be with the patient throughout each day.

## CHATTERBOXES

There is a line that is often crossed when a patient is the topic of 'passing discussions' in a public setting within the facility. Despite new and interesting information that might be on the table, it's your job to fight the propensity for what can be considered gossip in the workplace. 'Gossip' implies an air of negativity around the conversation, but what it really is, is speaking in a way that does not protect the patient's privacy.

## HIPAA

We have an obligation to maintain the standards of the Health Insurance Portability and Accountability Act (HIPAA), which outlines a set of national standards for protecting health information. While it is a necessity for health providers to transfer information conveniently, a guideline must account for the responsible use and the security of the information, so that no one can use it for any unintended purposes—whether beneficial or detrimental to the client. There are penalties for failing to comply with HIPAA, which can be found on the Department of Health and Human Services (HHS) website.

Take heed: be careful about what you allow to leave your lips, and under what conditions you do it. It's not always something you'll see coming. Recently, I answered the phone on a residential floor, as I was sitting at the nursing station. It was a number not from within the facility, and usually I wouldn't answer such calls, because it's mostly just a series of questions I don't have the answers to. If not that, it is a request to look for someone to pass along a message, which cuts into time that I don't want to use unproductively if I don't know where to find that person. In other words, it's too much pressure. However, given that the number kept calling, I gave in. It was a patient's son who called to check in on his mother's status.

I gave him the general information: "She's doing well, I saw her for therapy today."

He was happy to hear that, but wanted to know more. He asked, "Is she on oxygen? What medications is she taking?"

Before he went further, I told him I was unable to provide medical information, and even more so, that I couldn't do it over the phone. I understood that it devastated him, because he couldn't visit her at the time, but I knew it wasn't my position to take the risk of sharing more than what I could, legally.

Yes, HIPAA applies to family members and friends, too. With the patient's permission, I could have given more information over the phone, but she wasn't awake to do so, so it was still true that I didn't know all the necessary details. Therefore, it was best to redirect him to someone who did and could be of greater help.

There are cases in which you get to know family members very well, even by name and face. They will ask you questions about things in relation to their mom, grandma, uncle, or whoever. In these cases, I advise you to share only what is within your scope of practice that relates to the patient's therapeutic plan of care. If you know they are actively involved and are using the information to implement whatever means of care for the patient's quality of life, then it is reasonable to share. However, if you chat with them about a strategy that's been working for them in their communication, and the conversation leads to something medical, there is a wide range of possibilities that when you start talking, you may overstate or complicate what would be best communicated by the patient's physician or the nursing supervisor. The same goes for physical therapy, or any other care provider. I make it a habit to be "not too sure" to encourage family members to ask the appropriate professional.

## If I May Ask...

While we're thinking of ways to keep other people out of our patients' business, we also have to exercise a level of inhibition when dealing with our patients. While we're all becoming friends, there's a limit to what is appropriate to ask. For example, it's not too outrageous to inquire how many children a patient has—actually it's a common discussion in speech therapy for long-term memory, etc—but it may be a step beyond their comfort level for you to ask about the reason for their divorce. If that has left his or her long-term memory, it's a great blessing, so leave it that way.

Our patients learn to trust us. Be careful not to bring up information your patient shared with you in privacy in front of other staff. If the patient is alert and notices you doing this, they may lose their trust in you and not share information about their private life with you again.

As much as you want to care for the patient's privacy, do note that you have a right to yours as well. Patients will sometimes ask questions you may not be comfortable with: your age, your marital status, etc. While they will typically mean no harm, you have every right to tell them you don't want to share.

Questions may arise innocently, but care and attention to the appropriateness of the conversation between yourself and the patient is crucial. I did an externship once. The clinical supervisor left two other students and me high and dry to treat a patient for speech therapy. She didn't want to be present for the sessions because the patient was especially interested in her because of their relation to one another linguistically and culturally. He was cognitively impaired and his pragmatics—in terms of inhibition—were not all too great. He asked constantly about her marital status and complimented her on her physical appearance.

Her delegation of the tasks was, to us as students, a questionable solution, but I came to understand the reasoning very well. His behavior crossed over into a new realm beyond the patient's and provider's right to privacy. It is, in fact, very important to let as many necessary ears as possible hear these stories, especially if it crosses the line from innocent questioning to pursuing sexual innuendos or behavior.

## Inappropriate Patient Sexual Behavior

Inappropriate patient sexual behavior (IPSB) is encountered more times than one can keep track of in the rehab or senior care setting. It happens to rehab therapists, nurses, and other staff. According to Judith Dicker Friedman, an occupational therapist and article writer on EL Direct Home Care, the best way to approach these behaviors is in a non-judgemental and re-directive way. While there is an understanding that all beings have the right to sexual expression, it is not okay for the staff member or therapist to allow the behavior to continue. The staff member should be assertive and state the consequences of continued behavior. The careful delegation of the patient's case to another trained professional can reduce the chances of this behavior continuing.[1]

## PANTS... OR NO PANTS

Now, it goes without saying that you're in someone's home when you work in the SNF. It's just about impossible to make it through a full day without catching someone in their birthday- or half-birthday suit.

We intend to avoid cleaning, dressing, and bathroom times; however, if you start your work before 9 AM, it's likely that you'll find your patient still in bed, and, at best, only halfway decent for your arrival. While it's essential to knock first and pull a curtain when needed, the reality is that most people aren't especially shy. You'll be shocked at how eager a patient can be to converse with you during their morning routine or nude afternoon-lounge. At other times, he'll decide in the middle of your session, while it's just you and him, that he needs assistance to get to the toilet... immediately. This is one of those 'not-my-job' kind of things you just do, because if he's left to his own devices, things will be way worse than dealing with a naked person for two seconds.

When dealing with the cognitively impaired and behavioral patient, disrobement may be a habit that helps the patient to cope. Offering to redress, a change of clothes, a towel, or a blanket is just ethical. When this doesn't work, I have to be frank—you have limited options. Therapy is hard to take seriously in these cases, but your 30 minutes wind down very quickly while wrestling a shirt onto a crazed and combative elderly woman. While there are a few ways around this problem, it's most important to make the best use of the time to answer the question of why they do it, rather than to make them stop. It can be a response to temperature, pain, or something sexual. The previously discussed approach to inappropriate patient sexual behavior does not work with these patients. Despite that this expression is allowed to some extent, it can also be an interruption to the general population if they do this in, say, the main dining room. It can disrupt therapy potential as well, because they are unable to focus with clothing on. You can, to the best of your ability, use it as an opportunity for pragmatic training and, otherwise, ensure their greatest possible level of comfort, even if that means that they complete treatment time naked.

The SNF—any health care setting, really—is a bad place for the prude. Between the cussing and the regular R-rated displays, it's sort of laughable when we consider how many off-the-wall things happen in one day. Sometimes, however, it is really necessary for the patient's health and management to discuss certain topics, immodestly while maintaining a straight face about it. A voice in the back of my head still whispers, "This isn't normal," but my day keeps moving as if it is. They always did say in grade school if someone makes you nervous, picture them in their underwear. Well, in healthcare, if this ever makes you nervous, just picture them with clothes on.

**CHAPTER FOOTNOTES**

[1]Dicker Friedman, Judith. "Inappropriate Client Sexual Behavior Training." EL Direct Home Care, n.d. https://www.eldirecthomecare.com/inappropriate-client-sexual-behavior.html.

# 18

# DUE DILIGENCE

*A Guide to Surviving Your Patients*

I figuratively place my feet into my patients' shoes so far as to be at my own dinner table, having only eaten a few bites of my food—perhaps because my mind is on something else. Sometimes, I would eat in the driver's seat of my car in between sites—very fast—because I felt rushed going between facilities, with no time for a break. Of course, I noted my own prolonged mastication, delayed trigger, and cough during a meal, and I had the opportunity to laugh about it and still eat what I wanted, because nobody was taking it away from me. Aside from that, I wouldn't have passed my own test; go figure—I didn't have to.

A new resident, unaccustomed to food that's chopped up or manipulated, may love to know the intricate details of why the steak his family had packed up and delivered for him is not really the best choice for him to eat. His family may also have some questions or comments, along the lines of, "But he's not choking," even though 30 minutes later, he's only made it through three bites, he's not full, and certainly hasn't received the needed nutrients from the meal to help him improve his overall status. You can consider it a work of constant effort to keep everyone around you and around the patient on the same page.

There are those who are especially peculiar. Perhaps they believe healthcare is a scam, that their 30 minutes with you fills your wallet with gold, or—my favorite—that they don't need therapy. Then there are those that think you are a magician, a lucky charm, or some kind of goddess. Others may think you are their secretary or intern. They may ask about things that aren't within your scope or talk about topics they had better save for prayer or at least a mental health specialist. Sometimes all of this outweighs all the resources and time you have to provide therapy to them. When you get to know your patients a little, you'll know how to follow up.

There are the patients who make you run your full daily goal of steps on your fitness app, from their bedside to the kitchen, to the pantry, to the nursing station, and to the chapel to beg for mercy. Then there are those who would prefer to spend the entire session slowly accommodating to one exercise or one food item, which they may not even master in the allocated time. I swear, there is hardly any in-between. Neither is it all bad or all good, unless a patient solemnly refuses to do anything you ask of them. You'll get several patients who are just disinterested.

That being said, even after you've mastered the ins and outs of making it through your day as your building's SLP, there are still challenges related to communication that you're sure to come by. The journey through therapy is sometimes rocky, and a landmine can go off at any moment. You stay the course because there is a potential that the patient might achieve, and you feel that you can help them get there. What about when you don't feel like you can get them there? Obviously, if your skill level is the reason for this, there are a wealth of individuals that can help you get along to a point at which you're comfortable. Don't turn away a patient because you don't have all the answers yet. If you don't try, who will?

## THE CYCLE

It's not always the answer to stay the course, especially if you aren't willing to change anything about your approach. I have been at the point of just going to work to follow the same routine: clock in, see Patient X, stay for 30 minutes, do oral motor exercises, do pharyngeal exercises, give him a cookie, give him water, leave, place orders, document, notify the staff. See Patient Y. Repeat.

This is a quick way to demotivate your patient and yourself. You may not be communicating enough. You may not be putting yourself in other people's shoes as often as you can. You're skipping many questions. I've been there. I became discouraged and impatient when I was forcing something that wasn't working. As a result, my abilities as a clinician faltered.

When that happens, consider the domino effect it has on the patients you see. Your patients most especially deserve a good start and finish with you. At the very least, communicate with them about their day and how they're feeling. You have several more boxes to check off on your daily visits, but your patient may have other plans. When you treat them as people, you recognize how their feelings and physical imbalances get in the way sometimes. It may get in your way, too, and that's a daily pill you swallow. You must instead seek to achieve a greater quality in your connection with the patient in order to serve them better. It will not only gain you trust and leeway into treating them effectively, but will immensely reduce your propensity to become frustrated by the therapeutic process.

## THE MARATHON TO DISCHARGE

This is one setting in which your decisions as a clinician are mostly autonomous. During your CFY, you may confer with your supervisor or rehab director about various people you treat; it is ultimately your decisions that count the most, because you see the patients for the greatest amount of time, and you know them best. While your higher ups may run you a list of questions, you may realize they tend to just lead you to your own water rather than pouring the bottle down your throat.

Let's say you begin your due diligence by completing a clinical evaluation with the individual, using Tidbits (chapter 9), and you've determined what his needs and reachable goals are. However, it turns out your patient is not the perfect candidate.

What is the perfect candidate, anyway? Well, the perfect candidate has:

- No cognitive deficits.
- No internal illness.
- No more than 1 year of history of the presenting problem.
- No mental health or depressive issues.
- He or she is self-motivated.
- Staff and family who are involved and knowledgeable about the presenting problem.

The only thing you have to worry about is treating for his speech- or swallowing-related diagnosis.

If only you lived in a perfect world.

Your patient hates oral motor exercises, but you expected him to achieve at least 75% success with isometric tongue protrusions against resistance. Now what? He's over you and laughs at you when you're looking silly as ever, holding your tongue out to cue him for this exercise for the hundredth time. Poor you.

It's really easy to understand why this is not our patients' favorite activity, although it's ours, because we know the world of difference it makes for the muscle groups involved. We know the effects it's bound to have when done correctly, and it's so straightforward, even a baby can do it. How does that help the patient who has already decided it's useless?

It doesn't. It's almost never worth it to force it. If it's not done correctly, it does virtually nothing for the patient and frustrates you in the process. There's always the consideration of a passive form of the exercise, but that also proves to be significantly less impactful on the patient's function.

It might not be a bad idea, in this case, simply to let it go and work on something else. Perhaps you don't have to drop the goal entirely, but you need to approach it differently. If you are doing oral motor exercises because the patient has mastication issues, perhaps you can train them with increasingly tougher consistencies; nutritive work is just as good, if not better, than non-nutritive work. If the problem is with oral transport or clearance, perhaps a variety of compensatory strategies could be helpful. In combination with these, you may consider using focused attention to each portion of the phase in question, especially doing tongue placement and sweeping and strengthening where oral residue usually collects.

Where cognitive deficits are considered (and they often will be) you have a limited range of options. Contrary to popular belief, that's not yours to ponder and pout about. I have done so in the past, and I promise it isn't useful. A real survival tactic is to reduce everyone's overall burden, including the patient's, the caregiver's, and your own. Working miracles is the Lord's job. Yours is to educate and document. When you think a patient is just not agreeing with the therapy, you must make a decision. In this case, you may choose to 'abort mission,' but never before you do your due diligence.

Here are a few examples of therapy courses that led to discharge before my patients met all their goals.

# STORY TIME WITH ZEKE
## Healthcare—a Scam?

I once had a patient (for HIPAA purposes, we'll call him Zeke). He had a diagnosis of schizophrenia and had made claims of abuse by healthcare workers. Zeke was impossible, a tad less so when his brother was around to help care for him. By impossible, I mean that Zeke thought so deeply about each question, it was confusing to tell if he didn't know how to answer, or if he just didn't want me to know the answer. The questions were generally orientation-based or based on hobbies and interests to prompt expressive language. Most of the session's time, instead, went into me repetitively answering questions like, "Why does this matter, anyway? Why do you need to know that? How do you even know that about me?" I soon realized that it was a mechanism he put together to obscure his difficulties in responding, and I assured him it was okay to make mistakes or to ask for help. He was very resistant to new ways of overcoming those difficulties because of an unreasonable anxiety, which was not under his control. I had explicitly established my presence, purpose and intentions, but Zeke never really allowed me enough leeway to treat him. He didn't understand why I was there, and he unfortunately did not trust me, nor wanted me there. After several weeks of educating and motivating, I ended the case without having achieved much progress.

Do you think I did my due diligence? Explain.

_____

_____

_____

What else could I have done?

_____

_____

_____

(I am no stranger to correction, nor do I fear it. Perhaps you feel that I missed something. I always look back on cases and consider that there may have been more options than what I considered. Ideally, you'll cover all your bases before discharge, but it has happened days after a discharge that the patient perked up or a light bulb turned on suddenly.)

I think I did my due diligence with Zeke. Decreased motivation is one strong indicator that therapy is going downhill or, at best, reaching a plateau just as quickly as the therapy course begins. His psychological disorder was a drawback to therapy intervention, and seemingly it was not under control. It deserved more attention before the speech and cognitive rehabilitation were to be even remotely successful. In my opinion, I exhausted the options available, remained open to listening and answering questions, and geared the therapy activities to things he identified as his interest areas. In the end, he was clearly disinterested in any continuation of this intervention, and that was that.

# STORY TIME WITH SAM
## *Language Barriers*

Sam spoke very little English, and I knew not one word in his language. Such is the plight of the SNF settings I worked in-we had limited access to translation services in such situations. Sam's son was handy and usually present at the bedside when I came to see Sam for therapy. His son translated, but not well. Somewhere during our ethics course in graduation school, I'm sure we learned the dangers of using family members as translators. But the options were narrow. After I'd explained to the son in every way possible-aside from obtaining the actual fiberoptic endoscopic evaluation of swallowing (FEES) video-what the problem was, what we had to try to avert the damage, and how exactly the exercises should have been done, I truly didn't know what else to do.

As I continued to look for new ways to cue Sam and reword the information for his son, his son kept asking me about his broken arm and arm sling, his time in physical therapy, and about his term of stay in the facility. These questions outweighed the questions about swallowing by far, and I came to a point that I was fed up. Responding with "I have no idea" didn't reduce the son's inclination to ask me such questions. I'd already redirected him to the appropriate people to ask about his other medical and therapy needs, and somehow he still didn't get the answers he was looking for.

I didn't allow this to be the basis of discouragement, even though it was very annoying. I drew pictures for Sam, I modeled the exercises at every angle, I walked slowly through conversations with the little English Sam had, and I used a staff member that spoke a similar dialect of his native language to explain the precautions to him. It didn't seem like Sam was making any gains-at all. After several more weeks, I called it quits and allowed the thin liquids in a 'free water protocol' sort of directive.

Do you think I did my due diligence? Explain.

_____

_____

_____

What else could I have done?

_____

_____

_____

I don't think I did my due diligence with Sam. The language barrier should not continuously present at a level like it did, and it was my responsibility to look into more professional ways to handle that. Creativity was not the answer in this case, as none of the mural art that I painted hoping to inspire him was working. Sam would have benefitted from something more well-tested and guaranteed to get the job done, like an Iowa Oral Performance Instrument (IOPI) trainer. We had nothing like that in my setting, but I also didn't advocate for it at a time that I could have. I had the fault, also, of leaving potentially useful material out of my reach, so it put us at a reduced propensity for success.

# STORY TIME WITH PEARL
## Opa!

Pearl was a sweetheart from what I could gather, but her daughter was a bit of a terror. Pearl was over the age of 90 with a diagnosis of Parkinson's that had clearly advanced to a point past which her daughter could care for her. She was severely contracted, confused, and barely verbal.

Although Pearl had been on a PEG tube for a number of years, her daughter still fed her by mouth. This led to several instances of aspiration pneumonia. During her time at our SNF, Pearl's daughter finally accepted that oral feeding was no longer an option. But there were other issues. I had also been seeing Pearl for speech therapy to increase her communication activity. We tried several types of stimulation for her to speak-as much as we could think of. Music, gestures, you name it.

At the end of the therapy, it was still only during spontaneous instances that she would verbalize something loud and clear. Overall, though, Pearl was barely intelligible. I informed her daughter that we would discontinue the service, and this information was very difficult for her; she expressed her disappointment aggressively. On one occasion, she told me I didn't know what I was doing, and that I didn't like white people. Before long, Pearl and her daughter were on their way out the door-this was for more reasons than the speech therapy, but certainly, she had her qualms about this.

Do you think I did my due diligence? Explain.

_____

_____

_____

What else could I have done?

_____

_____

_____

I believe I did my due diligence with Pearl, with the help of her daughter—as loopy as she was. Speech therapy really relies on including as many parts of the patient's life, likes, and traditions as you can. With Pearl's daughter, we found music in her native language and for the holiday she loved most, I began calling her "Ma" because she only responded to that name and not her given one, and her daughter would engage her in their native language conversationally, and although I didn't understand, I could appreciate that she was more responsive in this language than she was in English, though she spoke both. Her daughter wasn't wrong in implying that she could speak. The thing was that her only motivation to speak was her daughter. The little that she did resulted from a significant decrease in overall function. Pearl was, in the doctor's words, ready to die soon. This must have been an immensely difficult moment for Pearl and her daughter, but after the two months we had spent together, I didn't feel like there was much wiggle room left for me to intervene.

## FAMILY FIRST

Let's not forget that due diligence is hardly ever complete without the loved ones of the patient you are seeing for therapy. Where you falter in understanding or run short of ideas to motivate someone, the family is, many times, the answer. Sometimes, families don't visit as often as they should. As much as you can keep them in the circle, do it! They are the most important and need to understand something new their family member is going through. Your introduction opens a path to listening and applying the information you give them. Some families you will never meet, and some will give you honorary membership into their tight-knit circle. It has its perks; I've once had a patient's daughter make me Mangu! (A Dominican dish of plantain mash served with egg.)

There are drawbacks with family. You read in this chapter about some of my experiences—good and bad. Sometimes, you'll be sought out to clarify and apologize for something that was not your fault or was beyond your decision-making abilities. Some families will try to scare you and insist that your recommendations are not considerate of who the patient is and what they need. Sometimes, they aren't wrong, but once you are able to have those conversations, progress can be made. It's much better when they know you by face and name and trust that you have their loved one's best interest at heart.

Due diligence is not just checking off a bunch of boxes. Although a discharge from therapy in the long-term setting is not a 'goodbye' but most likely a 'see you later,' it is a thoughtful and comprehensive end to a journey with someone that you've hopefully built a meaningful rapport with.

I used to respond jokingly to residents who greeted me with, "I haven't seen you in..." or, "It's been a while," with, "That's a good thing. It's a bad day if I've got to come check up on you."

While friendships may last, bring this portion to a close with just as much care as you opened it. Ask yourself the question of how the patient is going to meet their feeding- or communication- related needs without you. It's an unspoken goal, but one that requires thought and planning. You will not be able to provide the level of care you did during the therapeutic process, and you have to turn it over to family, nursing, and other staff. Do you think that you've put in your due diligence to ensure the patient is at their highest possible level?

# Part Five

## TAKING CARE OF YOURSELF WHILE CARING FOR OTHERS

# 19

# ACHOO!

## *A Guide to the Flu*

It's extremely interesting that I am writing this chapter, and most of this book, amid the COVID-19 crisis. Coronavirus is taking over everything, and I can only think about what my facility had endured, and how we expected it to be alleviated by extreme training on handwashing. We have had lasting effects on the way we do everything—while for some, ongoing news about the numbers of those affected by this global pandemic has only made them more freakishly aware of germs.

Before delving into that, I would advise that you never go to work sick—pandemic or no pandemic. In the colder months, take extra precautions to avoid sniffing in those loving germs people bring with them when they come to the facility. Masks, gloves, and frequent handwashing and sanitizing do a great deal of good when it's flu season. I advise that you get the flu shot simply because we SLPs can't avoid working with the mouth, and we are often up close when a patient decides it's time to cough. I've been at the other end of the projectile secretions (even food!). It sucks. I have two poor habits: touching my face and biting my nails. Working in a nursing home hasn't quite broken these habits, even though they've been bent. I have new, weird sensory reactions to things that are wet or sticky, especially if it's on my hands. Since my immune system has proven to be ironclad, I have little fear of getting sick, but even I have become more intentional in my daily behavior to avoid the unnecessary spread of germs.

## FLU SEASON ON STEROIDS

Our facility experienced the biggest quarantine I could have ever imagined—just as the COVID-19 pandemic became common news. One patient caught what they thought to be the flu, and before long, the entire sixth floor consisting of 40 beds was under lockdown. I remember hearing the news that the facility would only allow necessary visits, and rehab could just forget about treating those patients. Rehab—not seeing as many patients as possible? Must be something serious...

Before the true resolve of what seemed to be a localized problem, came the gigantic wave of the groundbreaking world-wide-spreading virus. It was hard to tell where one ended and the other began. In the beginning, COVID-19 was handled the same way our flu quarantine went. We were in for so much more than we expected... Soon after one floor closed, the second, then the third was suspected of having some cases of high fever. The facility experienced a dramatic census turnover. Many patients were temporarily hospitalized, and many others could not withstand the symptoms and died in-house. I wore that damned surgical mask over my N-95 for hours on end, breathing my own hot carbon dioxide. I struggled to model exercises to my patients. Having extensive verbal interaction eventually changed my body temperature. My patience was thinning even quicker than our population of residents.

COVID 2020—it's fit to refer to it as an era—has been no easy feat for nursing homes, especially those in New York City. The initial wave was nothing less than a massacre, and from the standpoint of the staff in the facility, getting up and going to work was no longer just clockwork. For myself, it was a daily, literal headache and my emotions were constantly off balance. It wasn't odd for anyone to well up with tears at any random point of the day when the weight of it all came bearing down.

What did this mean for the facility? Well, at first, they wanted to keep things as rigid as possible, more to protect the patient population than to protect the staff. This was noticeable when they sent us rehab therapists to the affected floors to treat barely viable patients with known diagnoses of COVID.

Our staff tried to protest, as many were calling in sick. We'd gotten wind of several patient and staff deaths, and for those advanced in age or with other health issues, it was a scary thing to manage. We were denied full body suits, and instead given thin, flimsy disposable gowns as personal protection equipment (PPE) in the climax of the pandemic—just to be offered the full body suits one week later. I still wonder why they had the change of heart.

I happened to cover at other facilities, because a few from our agency had tested positive for the virus. At first, in the absence of a fever, many were still mandated to work. No one received hazard pay. Later, they required symptoms to be managed at home for a week. There was a transition from the use of agency paid time off (PTO) to state-funded sick time. My manager texted me each and every morning at 7 AM to inquire about any symptoms, to the point at which I wanted to scream aloud, "I'm not sick, I'm just extremely sad!" Yes, I took some time to manage that, as well.

With advancements in biotechnology, we could finally have in-house testing for all staff and the dwindling patient population. The facility handled most symptoms in-house, unless it worsened to the extent of requiring hospitalization. Appointments and visits were totally canceled, aside from necessities such as dialysis. By June, our building was COVID-19-free. Still, patients were tested twice monthly and staff twice weekly. The world was opening up again, and we were slowly implementing ways to reconnect patients with their families and preparing for a return to some normalcy of things.

Flu season, and general precautions around the medical setting, will literally never be handled the same. My clairvoyance tells me that masks and timed quarantines upon admission or readmission from hospitals will become routine. Even though we've progressed to a point at which people have instantaneous test results and can be confirmed as having a negative status, our entire system requires high levels of precautions of using masks, engaging in socially distanced activities and meetings, limiting personnel, and adapting schedules. However, what remains the most important precaution—personal hygiene—is becoming less strictly monitored.

All this being said, what has it meant for us as speech-language pathologists?

## A THREAD

### PPE

Masks are now the norm. This means speech and swallow therapies are 20 times harder, especially with those who need the visual models to complete exercises. While some creative soul has designed a mask that has a transparent barrier, it is not welcome at my facility. If this is not a reasonable option for you either (consider that it does not have the N95 or KN95 protection), pictures and videos as visual stimuli may suffice along with passive techniques and gestures.

### Low Caseload

This has been the hardest pill to swallow. With the progression and resolve of the virus in my facility, has come a wave of high and low census. At some points, patients entered the facility at almost the same rate as they had previously left—on stretchers or in body bags. The new patients were most often COVID positive, and many were short-term. As my time at the facility was ending, most patients had returned home, and their beds were left empty, with no new patients to bring the census back to normal. My caseload in August was down to five people, while I was used to seeing 12–15 on a regular day. Considering that the fluctuation of caseloads is high in the SNF without COVID, screening and picking up in-house is typically a viable option to keep things afloat. That option has been used and overused to the point that it is moot. Many of the serviceable patients were no longer with us, and I'm sure that's still the case. It's interesting that the long-term PEG feeders and those with severe cognitive impairments seemed to have fared better than others through the pandemic. Before I left, I did get some value in doing more speech and language pickups, but what is to come seems extremely bleak for the SNF. If you've already accepted a CFY in a SNF, ensure that they will account for your hours to provide full days of work, if that's what you need. It may also be worth your while to find out if there are options for working in between facilities. If you are already in a position and seeing decreased hours, find out if your agency offers a Paycheck Protection Program (PPP).

### Referral

Because of the steep decline in the availability of outsourced services for patients, you must expect some pushback during your referral process. Skilled providers are slowly returning to the surface, and patients who have had to wait to receive attention for vision, dental, and other services are finally getting what's overdue. Anything requiring a trip to the hospital is re-thought twice or more, because the risk of contracting COVID is considerably higher for someone who leaves a virus-free and controlled facility. That even meant no MBS studies for some time, so our weaning programs were progressing more slowly or completely halted. Getting around the middleman where possible is still necessary. This means more conversations with nursing staff, phone meetings when needed, and just revising your plan if all else fails.

Do not take lightly how much this experience has changed healthcare many personal lives. The survival tips of this chapter are to move with an extra pep of positivity in your step and to be patient with others and even more with yourself. Stay planned, prepared and prayed up, because we do not know what is to come.

# 20

# PARIS, ANYONE?

## *A Guide to Taking Time Off*

Given all we've talked about, it's no secret that the SNF will offer an experience that is in equal parts rewarding and exhausting. Benefit does not come without burden. It is the living definition of "you reap what you sow." When you put in the work, the results can be beautiful. The experience is not all the glitter of academia—no confetti at the end of every milestone, no sparkling A when your hard a** work ethic gets the job done right. Hardly ever a real "thank you" will come your way, but you'll know you're good when no one's stepping on your toes or chasing you down for late reports.

To thrive, you must exercise some self-care. While this applies to daily living (I am an advocate for frequent and extravagant self appreciation), once in a while, you should definitely step it up a notch. It's during that wishy-washy summer, when I didn't know what the heck was happening with my life or my finances, that I somehow found a way to travel. It has since been my best companion. I think about it when I'm not working...

Ah, who am I fooling? I've looked for plane tickets on the clock before.

I find all the ways people manage to travel while on the job fascinating. Even in the middle of the COVID-19 crisis, people are getting on planes and experiencing the world. I have to be completely honest: a part of what's made travel so big for me is the need to get away from the stress. This is my personal perspective, and I understand that it's not the only way to view this setting or this field. In my experience, stress has often taken a front seat. It's affected my physical and mental health, and while I feel like I always came out on the other side stronger and better than before, it was undeniable that I needed an outlet.

The responsibilities of working in a place such as a SNF can be extremely tolling, even if you handle stress well. Apart from understanding the process of palliative care, you tend to run around like a chicken with its head cut off to be productive, you have to defend yourself and your recommendations constantly, and look at a computer screen until you can see each

TATTLETALES OF A SPEECH-LANGUAGE PATHOLOGIST

pixel as though they are grains. Other areas that can drain you include: the near-constant demand for your subsequently divided attention, the burden of responsibility for things you cannot control, and the personal consequences of patients not meeting the potential you envision for them. I can go on and on about how necessary it is to have your own mental health in check to handle this kind of position. Especially if you don't have other people in your building that do what you do, or your supervision is minimal or affectionately detached—i.e., your supervisor does not care about your success—this can all get very rough very quickly.

Some people don't ever take time off. They just go on working—maybe for two or three years, if their vacation days roll over. Every week, five, six, or even seven days, they work. Side hustles and all, because that's what SLPs are known for. I am a hard worker, but by no means a workaholic. It gets a bit personal, but my mother and I have so much negative history that stemmed from her being a workaholic. By drowning yourself in work, personal connections with your family and loved ones are affected much more strongly than you may immediately notice.

My advice is not to work less, less hard, or even to take time off. Everyone's priorities will be different and valid. On my first vacation, I thought whoever's idea PTO was—I worship him. I went ahead and celebrated the end of my CFY with my second paid vacation, an 18-day solo trip to eastern Europe and the United Kingdom. I literally read the congratulatory text message on receiving my New York State (NYS) license while tipsy at a party in Greece. Shrug. I also made it to Africa twice in the same calendar year, which were such important and meaningful experiences for me as a black person.

My wanderlust grew to be bigger than myself, and sometimes bigger than the job. I've taken risks, and I would be lying if I said they weren't rewarding. The world is beautiful, and I have no thought of stopping traveling any time soon. Taking time off to travel has been my saving grace; it has pulled me from deep points of depression and gives me something to look forward to persistently. When you speak to people of the daily ins-and-outs of working, you realize life passes faster than you will ever be ready for it to. A speech-language pathology job may never make you rich, though it can make you financially comfortable. Your wealth is in mental health, and I can't stress that enough.

Taking PTO is not always so straight-forward. In fact, depending on the agency you work for, it can be damn near impossible to get the time you want exactly when you want it. The best advice that I have is to plan and communicate things in advance. Where your agency may only require two weeks' notice of your PTO, giving them two months or more has typically been more beneficial for me. With even that much notice, it isn't guaranteed and can become a strain on your vacation plans if you've already begun spending money on it.

If your agency is anything like the one I worked for, the network is small; so finding someone to replace you can be a tedious exercise for your manager. If you work directly within a facility, I couldn't tell you for a fact, but I imagine this being more difficult if they must outsource services. Either way, where you can, make this process as smooth as possible by setting the stage in advance of requesting your time. Though it is your right and responsibility to yourself, your job thinks of PTO as a gift and privilege, instead. Show them that you take care of that privilege by being considerate in any way you can see fit. If things are especially strenuous for your leaders, or you've called out several times before planning a vacation, it might not be the best time to ask—just saying.

It's always a good idea to offer a little extra where you can to sweeten the deal on your ideal vacation. In the past, I've given up holidays to leverage my PTO request for the week following the holiday. I've covered additional hours on top of my own to 'help out' when other staff were vacationing or sick. I've seen to it that my paperwork and other responsibilities were up to date and in good standing and that my caseload was at a manageable level, meaning that the rehab director wouldn't be bothered to decrease hours or look for additional help to cover everything. I've offered to ease the transportation needs of per diem staff that wouldn't take my facility because it was far away from a subway train.

I'll admit that you should take my advice in the way of taking time off with a grain of salt. You can do all of this and still run into a hardship when it is time to take your vacation. You may have the most manageable caseload and still be given hell because your agency doesn't want to find you coverage (or they just don't want you to take the time off). I've been there. It wasn't easy to see Africa twice in one year with a full-time job. I did everything I could to get my behind on a plane peacefully, and it still wasn't enough. Ultimately, I took the time that I needed at the risk of getting into a serious bind with my company leaders and potentially losing my job.

I don't recommend doing things my way and demanding time that isn't already determined to be yours. Instead, review what your needs are in advance and communicate your plans to your agency, company, facility—what have you—as soon as you know of them. An emergency time-off is a completely different ball game, and should not be taken lightly by yourself or the people you work for. Don't hesitate to communicate this need as exactly what it is: something that needs an immediate response. If your mental health, physical health, or family is at stake, I think the right thing to do is to prioritize that. If and when the time comes, you will know what to do.

# 21

# AH, RETIREMENT

## *A Guide to Surviving... Long-Term*

Now, this part of the book isn't really a guide to survival, seeing as I'm just a little ahead of you. Perhaps you have been in the field for a longer time and are looking to switch over to a new setting. Or maybe you're just curious about what lil' ole me has to say, and that's fine too. I welcome everybody, especially to this portion of the text, because it's about one of my new favorite topics—money.

I have only just started learning what retirement even means. As I'm writing, I'm 26 years old, I have some savings, a few investments, and some big ideas. I can't really clearly imagine the rest of my career, but I vaguely hear rejoicing, clinks of wine glasses, precious metals rubbing against each other, and, for some reason, crying babies as faint as the forest song.

Realistically, when I see myself in the next 30 years, I won't even be practicing. Maybe I will be researching or developing a new technique. Maybe I'll lounge in bed, enjoying the passive income from my thriving practice and soaring stock investments. Perhaps my successful authorship will have me leave the field to travel and do journalism about foreign policies and their effects on the learning of young children with complex mental and physical illnesses.

The sky's the limit.

Whether you are in your first profession or making a new beginning, if you are under the age of 55, there are plenty of opportunities to plan adequately for your retirement. For some, retirement seems so far away; it's not too early to get the ball rolling in the right direction. In fact, if I knew diddly squat about retirement options or money before grad school... well, I might not have gone to grad school—yet. If I still chose to, I would have ensured I'd be in an immensely better position. I didn't question God when I had that year off after not getting into a program, but I do wish He had given me some more signs so I could have used that time better.

Fast forward months after the completion of my CFY, my agency invited me to open a 401k account. It was at that moment I realized I didn't even know what a 401k was. Would it tie me to this job longer than I wanted to stay? How much was enough to contribute? I had a mountain of questions, which took a couple additional months to figure out. I opened the account with some questions still unanswered, but sure enough that there was more to gain than to lose.

Even if you're in the SNF for what we'll call a "good time, not a long time," there is no benefit to turning down an opportunity for free money. Your 401k belongs to you, not to your job or agency. The company you work for can match up to 100% of your contribution. My employer match was much lower, but I can't complain when it's free. It'll be passively growing for virtually the rest of the time it's left untouched. You will never lose access to it, and it isn't taxed for as long as you wait to receive distribution, which means more gains for you over that course of time. Check with your employer about their vesting schedule, which will determine how soon you have access to the part of your assets that your employer contributed.

Your employer might not offer you a 401k. Other employer-sponsored retirement plans would be the 403b if you work for a non-profit or government-based company, or a thrift savings plan if you are military personnel or a civilian federal employee. It would probably not apply to you as a SNF professional, though.. If none of the above are available options, you still do not want to delay planning. You may choose to manage your retirement investments through a traditional or Roth IRA (individual retirement account). These are also tax-advantaged, and you will reap the benefits of years of investing into these sorts of accounts. Your options are wider and you are more in control of your investment decisions. It is worth it to consider this type of account whether or not an employer already sponsors one for you. When you want your money to grow, but need a more liquid option—i.e., you can't wait until you're 59.5 years old—there are brokerage accounts for that.

How do you know how much you will need? This is probably the hardest question you'll ask early on in your retirement planning. It is the start of a fairly long road; none of us really know what 30 years from now looks like. When you break down the question, you take into consideration some of the most important things you desire to achieve. Are you looking to buy a house? Do you want to open a practice? How big? How far below your means are you willing to live before and after your retirement? Do you want to travel in your retirement? Do you think that 30 years is a satisfactory length of time for you to complete your plan? Do you have or want to have children? No two people are equally matched on every possible question, but there's always a plan that can work for you. Where all else fails, adjustments can be made that work in your favor. Your options are literally limitless. It's all about what you are willing to learn, and how hard you are willing to work.

The second hardest question is, "What kind of investor am I?" which can be translated to, "How much risk can I handle?" Your 401k is considerably low risk. It's destined to grow, but more slowly and gradually than other types of investments, as most of your money is placed into mutual funds. Your '30-year' number is estimated based on your contribution and employer match, and may well turn out to be just in the ballpark of that number if nothing crazy happens, like the coronavirus. Will that be enough? Honestly, maybe not. It depends on what kind of retirement you want, but considering the significant number of people that come out of retirement for financial reasons, it seems sensible to come up with a less airtight sealed plan while you can afford to. With an IRA, you can diversify and take on much more risk, recommended with the advice of a financial professional.

If your situation is anything like mine, this is the most money you've made at one job. Somehow or another, I guess I was supposed to figure out exactly what to do on my own, without guidance. Turns out that it took almost two years to get on a sort of decent track. I sort of realized one day that I will not live forever, but I am—ideally—not going to work forever, either. There's a whole other generation of wealth that I can be responsible for, beyond taking care of myself in the here-and-now. My advice: seek guidance while you're still in school. If you're already out, get a planner and a financial expert right after you finish this chapter.

There is so much that speech-language pathology offers, not only to people of all ages with communication and swallowing disorders, but to us providers—emotionally, spiritually, and financially. On the hush-hush, I didn't want to accept the opportunity for the 401k, because it made me feel permanently stuck to my company. Hear this: when I started to dedicate my time to learning about business and investing, I knew for sure I was never going to be stuck in any company ever in life for any reason.

In my personal statement for applying to my graduate programs, I highlighted my interest in private practice, because it sounded good. I tend to my own special blend of things I want; and if it's not 100% in line with my idea, I'll find creative ways to make it a reality. What I was hoping to achieve, I'd never seen or heard of before—an original idea. While I still love the idea, I have a renewed sense of understanding of what private practice entails, why it is beneficial, and what financial expectations would reasonably accompany a 'great idea.' Further, I recognize that reinventing the wheel is not the only—or even the best—way to achieve success in a self-run business.

Whether or not you plan on building your entire career around the SNF setting, you will need to be a creative thinker and a bit of a risk-taker to get the utmost benefit of what you'll learn in your CFY and in the years that follow. Great opportunities are all around you, but they rarely just fall in your lap. You are the driver here. How can you remold what you've learned to generate more income? I don't care if you're happy with your salary; you have absolutely no reason not to want more. If the system you're employed in uses materials from a publicly traded company, you have a step in the door that others do not to make money on that knowledge. Were you specially trained with an objective test of some sort, and can you train others? Do it. I'll tell you a few secrets in the next chapter, but for now, just think about where this is all going.

I'm no finance guru by far, obviously. I have a lot more to learn about money, and about how to even drive this thing we call a career. I'm sure some of you feel the same way. Money is extremely fickle and risks are inevitable in building anything valuable. You could fall behind on your plans, and your priorities could change. I think that's okay. SLPs are known for doing a little too much of... well, everything! We are flexible and skilled enough to dip our feet in wherever the water seems cool. It's so tempting to take flight after you've gotten your wings, but for God's sake, let's stick to the basics, first.

That being said, good on you if you're already on the path to paying down debt. For those with student loans above $100k, we have some work to do. Know that this number is not as outrageous as it seems for any reason other than the American system for higher education being flawed in most ways, including financial cost. Your plan to free yourself from this debt comes from countless others who have done it. Perhaps your agency qualifies you for student loan repayment. Perhaps you work for a non-profit or government-based job and qualify for forgiveness through that. It's rougher for us medical SLPs than some of our peers in the school settings, who automatically apply for something like this. We then have to find more creative ways to overcome the debt that holds a piece of our check hostage in between its sharp teeth for what could be a couple decades after we graduate. Still, it's not impossible to find a solution. Unless you die, you have to pay for it. Oh, did I say that out loud?

Private refinancing is one recommended option for those who qualify for a better interest rate. This can be done for one federal or private loan, or a consolidated plan. It's generally meant to take control of the debt with a lower interest rate and monthly payment to eventually pay a lower total amount in the end.

No matter how you choose to do it, loan repayment is ongoing for more time than we'd really appreciate, but perhaps at some point it becomes muscle memory. At that given point, I'd say you should look into just how much your income can support your debt repayment—student loan or otherwise—and how it relates to your lifestyle and your future plans. Of course, you may not know everything you want in five plus years from now, but is it even enough right now? Do you have more than you need? Can you save or invest?

These kinds of questions precede those like: what kind of number do you think you need to live passively after the age of 65? Do you even want to work until you're 65? How much are you comfortable spending to receive a decent return on your investment to your therapy, your business, or your assets unrelated to SLP? Does the time you are giving to being an SLP allow you to manage other important areas of your life? Are you getting to the bag the right way?

I once was asked during a meeting with an old boss, prior to returning to school, "What amount of money do you need to make?"

I told him I didn't know. At the time, student loans were not a concern, I paid no rent, I had no car, and essentially no care in the world. I was a hard-worker for the hell of being a hard worker. I saw up to fourteen-hour days at two jobs with no plan whatsoever. I'm different now, because I have more financial responsibility, but I still have work to do to build my vision of the kind of life I'm planning for and how to prepare for it. I never said I was writing this book because I had it all figured out, by the way.

Two important things that I've learned are annual percentage returns and compounding. To get the very best out of any sort of investment, an early start is key to accessing both of these benefits. Come the time for retirement, you will look at a figure much grander than you could have imagined rewarding yourself with after all those years of hard work. Starting only a few years in advance, when you realize retirement should be just around the corner, will leave you with fewer options and can be a recipe for disaster if unplanned misfortune arises.

# 22

# THE SECRET

*A Guide to the Lies, so You Know the Secret to Success*

Think of all the things you have seen in your time as a student and compile that with all you've seen in a SNF so far. If you haven't been in one yet, just think about what you've read, or hold off on answering this question. What is the most jaw-dropping piece of information, jarring sight, experience, or realization that has stopped you in your tracks, made you retreat from thinking you knew everything and that you had a handle, and got you staring at yourself in the mirror, wondering if this is really where you belong?

```
_____
_____
_____
_____
_____
```

If you haven't seen it yet, know that this point will come. By answering this question, you prove you are steps ahead of the new-hire CFY that still thinks health care is all gold and glitter. Perhaps this moment will change everything you thought you'd come into the field for, and everything you'll do next. Most of all, what it will do is determine how ready you are to handle whatever is to be thrown at you next.

It will become your secret superpower.

## THE FIRST SECRET

The medical setting can be the sparkles and fluff you see in the pictures they use for advertisement on the websites—only on its most off day. These are days that you review and realize nothing crazy happened, no one yelled, and the sound of call bells were not piercing through the very surface of your skull. You saw your patients, you made your productivity, you billed, and you went home in peace.

I'm noticing that many of the books I open lately start with the 'lies' society tells you about subjects that seem quite straightforward. In this case, one lie is that your days will be anything as straightforward as this. In fact, you've found a jewel in the rough if your 'regular' isn't 'rowdy.'

Now, that's not a bad thing for me. I do well under pressure, and I get bored easily. For these reasons, I actually liked that something always required my attention. Productivity was a tasty piece of cake on most days, and juggling tasks was my favorite circus act. It might be the New Yorker in me, but I truly make peace with noise. Another person may scoff at this or any of the other points I present, and that's totally expected. Most people want to go to work and have a regular day. If you want to be a speech-language pathologist—whether in a SNF, a hospital, a school, a day-hab, or a home-based program—I discourage you to believe a regular day even exists.

That being said, I feel SNF speech-language pathologists and other staff bear an uneven weight of rowdiness compared to other settings. Hell, it's all of them combined. Considering all the antics brought from home, along with crazy cousin Mary who doesn't follow any of the visitation-hour rules and feeds your fragile patient like it's Thanksgiving every day, you might as well dust your feet off, put your picture on the wall, and join the family Kumbaya.

WIn the SNF, we're supposedly light years away from the practices of the school setting, but there are a few things that translate all across the board in this field. For instance, when it's 9:00 AM and you're trying to catch Mr. Roberts for 1st period, and he's in the gym instead of in your therapy session, I'm sure the feeling is just about the same. Then, to make up for lost time, you'll find yourself 'pushing-in' to an activity group later in the day.

On a serious note, this rough job setting can reveal an even rougher and tougher system destined to fail you if you don't know why you're there. I believe that's where I found my biggest pushback.

To succeed in a SNF, you need to be in touch with your sense of self, confident in your skills, and adamant about your ethics. I tell on myself in a way in Let's Get Literate when I write about 'creative documentation.' You'll need this skill especially, because you'll be mandated to save your facility's behind at some point. As discussed, these big detriments are not avoided by telling big lies, but instead by the most miniscule of things, like wording. A scale up from this, you may be tempted to mush and mold your justification for picking up a case that may not see much progress. Another scale up from that, you may be asked to bill five more minutes, just because. Not only do you find that these strategies rarely create any positive difference for your patients, but it also puts you to less use, less learning potential, and less time for yourself over repeated instances of this.

If five minutes doesn't seem like a lot, consider what I said about compounding in Ah, Retirement (chapter 21). Time is money. Five minutes more for 10 patients is almost an hour of your day. Over the course of a week, it is four hours. You were paid for this time (I hope— documentation time doesn't always pay) but what did you gain, otherwise?

Your patients are the gold and silver that you come to work for each morning, but I've had to ask myself sometimes: why do I feel like I'm not doing enough? I struggled for more than one year of my still very new career constantly feeling that I couldn't really get a grasp. I felt this should be the time of my life. Within myself, however, I was extremely unhappy with my choice to work in a SNF, and I questioned if the field of speech pathology had anything better to offer me.

Really, I was just losing momentum.

You too may come to a similar point. You'll feel drained, and not in the way that makes you feel you're doing a great job, even if you are. Many people will run you ragged with difficult behaviors and rude antics. Some days will pass slower than a drugged tortoise. You'll find yourself explaining something for the tenth time, while it's being heard as though it's the first. You'll sit your chin into the palms of your hands and mull over how many times better you expected a situation to go—but it just didn't. At those times, maybe you'll be inclined to withstand doubt and get the better of the circumstance. At least, that's what I did time and time again.

I did a lot of self-blaming for what I experienced on the job. Through many methods of reshaping my way of thinking, that has changed. I learned the hard way that great things aren't impossible nor rare. Doubt is natural, and it isn't always wrong. It is more valuable to explore it and find answers for it than to simply withstand it.

When your on-the-job set up isn't serving you, almost anything is difficult to appreciate. What is your work bringing to your purpose?

You came into the field hoping to achieve something. Save yourself first!

The web of lies you'll be told by the people that control money will hold on to you tighter than a juicy fly on something smelly in the summertime.

"But I work for an amazing company!" That's what I said, too. Consider, though, that these people secured their own bags first and left yours for last. It's nothing to do with you — it's just business.

More than two years after accepting my great opportunity with my great company that offered me everything under the sun, I know that a great company doesn't equal a great healthcare system or a great life. You are in charge of maneuvering that.

No, five minutes or even four hours won't throw off your Ph balance; and you may very well use that time wisely to service your patient in a useful and ethical way. My point is that what belongs to you will be taken if you don't have a firm hold on it. Your time is yours. So is your purpose.

I know it's so cliche, but knowing your 'why' will be key to walking through those doors each day to make a real difference in someone's life. When I felt negative about my job position, I didn't feel comfortable seeking the leadership of my peers or my supervisor. I felt alone. I didn't want my mentor to feel that I'd failed her years of leadership and reference letters, just for me to not appreciate it. Instead, I rolled around in lies—those that I was told and those that I told myself—in order to get comfortable in my workspace and to 'get used to it.' I knew what I needed to get through the day, but my thirst for knowledge and growth was stunted.

I did not have a 'why.'

Nearing the end of my time in a SNF, I no longer wanted to be a part of those lies. My truth was my peace of mind, writing this book, doing distance learning, and servicing other people who really needed my help.

## THE SECOND SECRET

Recently, I encountered a book called The ONE Thing by Gary Keller[1]. In it, I learned that another lie society tells is that we, as people, will learn to do extraordinary things by learning how to be extraordinary at everything. This is an alternative fact. If your experience has been anything like mine throughout academia and life in general, you were valuable because you were well-rounded. You did well in math, science, and art. You may even love the field of SLP because of how flexible and fluid it is. Considering myself a 'jack of all trades,' it was a gold mine for me. I wanted to do everything for every disorder across the lifespan.

I'm not really one to pay attention to celebrities or how much money they make, but, perhaps, if you think of the most successful and well-paid person you know within this field, you can tell me their area of focus, how long they've been practicing in it, and maybe even list a few articles or books with their name on it. I'll tell you that they didn't get there by being flexible.

While I was a student, I drove for three food delivery services, sold my soul to tutoring menacing elementary school children, corrected grad papers in the university writing center, bought my first DSLR camera, and went to work on all of it as well as I possibly could. The reality was that I needed to make some sort of living, but I also harped on a lifelong bad habit of doing too much. Pair this with hobbies I picked up, like doing Spartan races, paper mache, and circus aerial arts, I really didn't have any direction to help me meet my purpose.

This all went kapoot the moment I began my CFY. There wasn't, in my mind, any possibility of managing what was then 10 to 12-hour days between two facilities. My spirit wanted to, but my flesh was weak.

Weighing the importance of a social life and my job was irrelevant. I knew where my focus had to be after all I'd been through to get there. However, I knew that every Monday to Friday, 9 AM to 7 PM, with the last two hours primarily accounting for my paperwork (which I chose to be unpaid for to protect my productivity) was not a lifestyle I'd ever really thought I'd have, nor did I desire it. I broke promises to parents whose children I instructed in reading and writing because I just had no time to show up. Typically, when I left work, the sun was leaving or already gone, reminding me that my opportunity to do anything else with my day was also gone with it.

Apparently, it's not unusual to cry during drives home after a long day of work at the SNF when you're the only SLP on duty and the influx of admissions has been in multiples. It's no less anticipated to have this response when you're trained to extend yourself to many different things and then get trapped into one that's not always so fun.

At least in graduate school, I had options.

If I could, I would dissolve right here how much brain power it took me to get adjusted to my one thing. Coincidentally, the purpose of having one thing, is to do less brain work and more real work. It's to do the littlest thing you can do now to reach whatever your pinnacle or idea of success is. Think of it as a stepping stone to that great, big thing that seems unreachable.

## THE THIRD SECRET

With the 'one thing' philosophy, we recognize that multitasking is a moot tactic to enhance focus to create success. In the SNF, it seems almost impossible to avoid. You're constantly planning your next move, doing paperwork while your director is talking at you, and probably a million more things are on your plate. I like to think that although we are juggling plenty of tasks, we can only hold one of them at a time.

Procrastination is a bigger devil than multitasking when it comes to harnessing your one thing. If you put it off, you lose out on your ability to time block for adequate attention to your one thing. You might forget it. You aren't doing it religiously. Eventually, you find yourself some significant way down the line, not having achieved the greatness you intended to at the start.

Learning to say "no" will be the greatest gift you give yourself by the end of your fellowship. Again, your time is yours. Every moment you spend away from your 'thing' is lost to something else. This isn't to imply that other things aren't important; many of them are. But your priority is your thing. An alternative to "no" can be, "But I can do it by this given time..." or, "allow me to cross off X amount of things from my list first." This, in fact, improves your ability to show people how directed you are.

Notice when your willpower is at a high and when it is at a low. For instance, I know that whatever I do after lunch is far less momentous than what I handle in the early mornings. Therefore, I made it a point to get to the patients first, especially when notes were due or I expected diet changes. Paperwork didn't require the best of motivation, but my patients did. I constantly charged and recharged to give them the best of my service.

When you notice your willpower is being drained by your 'regular' run around, which can seem like a hamster wheel, you should re-evaluate your position and ask all the important questions that will ultimately divulge one thing you need to do to make something around you light on fire.

You can identify your 'one thing' strategy within any part of your life that is truly important to you. Hopefully, as a CFY, becoming an amazing SLP is a part of what you hope to achieve. Maybe you just want good, steady money—but if that's the case, I don't think you would or should be here reading this book. I'll write you another one specifically for that.

If you're here for the right reasons, you may find a 'thing' within your one thing. That particular patient or case throws you off your tracks, onto your toes! You find yourself researching more and more information to make sure you don't make any wrong moves, but also because learning feels rewarding again. You'll overcome the monotone (trust me, even 'rowdy' can become repetitive). Ask yourself: Where am I making a difference? Who else can I apply this to across my caseload, or even to my interactions around the building? Is it making me a little bit better every day? Does it relate to my why? Am I disciplined to see it all the way through?

Keller says that the path to great answers is great questions. The fourth secret is to never tire of asking more questions.

## THE FOURTH SECRET

Your practicum supervisor probably told you that you can never measure a patient's progress with a broad and vague goal. Don't cut yourself short with low-quality goals, either. What can you do right now to create intentional and immense results for yourself in a specified amount of time, so that you can be satisfied with your career, access your 'why,' and be financially secure and free?

But first come the fundamental questions. Maybe you can start with what's holding me back? Why am I not satisfied? Or what does 'satisfactory' even look like?

You know, for me, getting out of graduate school was a world war and a half. I was asking questions, but I was mostly pushing through to my light at the end of the tunnel. I knew where I could and could not handle setbacks. I was on a track with a vision, but obstacles came, as they always will.

My CFY was sort of an extension of this, but I felt ready for it. My jarring experience was much earlier—actually the first time I walked into the ICU at a local hospital where my mentor serves as the speech department director. The room was well lit, but the outlook for me was dark. An air-controlled room with a running ventilator attached to a patient with a tube that looked larger than you would imagine the throat was, laid out as if the grim reaper had already said his grace. I was just a volunteer. What I've experienced in the SNF as a licensed professional has never run me off my tracks in the same way. I'm not saying I always know what to do, but I always try to remember that the answers are not too far away from the right questions.

With time, the CFY became easy. Paperwork was just a way of life, and I rolled with the punches much more effortlessly than I did at the beginning. Literacy instruction and my social life regained some traction. Of course, I still had a lot to prove, but my CFY supervisor was letting up on the reigns as I became more confident and consistent with my responsibilities around my buildings, and as my documentation became more comprehensive.

Eventually, I slowed down and stopped asking questions. At that point, I just wanted to clock in, work, and clock out—nothing more, nothing less. I was signing my own paperwork and seeing myself through each day, so I didn't wait for people to tell me I was wrong or that they expected more of me. Ultimately, it was me who expected more. If you ever find yourself in this web of lies, believing that you have done too much or even just enough, that you've answered all the questions and passed the big test, I'm telling you—you're wrong. My survival tip to you: don't just seek to survive the CFY. The years following are even more critical. Consider and reconsider those questions, and adjust your focus as needed.

When I discovered a desire to travel, I thought that speech-language pathology couldn't travel with me. I came to a point—a low point... many low points, actually, before I started asking questions again. I asked myself what I really wanted. I asked God about the obstacles in my path. Then, I started asking for a new job and more pay. As I write, I'm asking, "What is the one thing I can do to self-publish and advertise this book to the curious souls approaching their start in the SNF and in this field, so I can successfully sell one million copies and retire on that income?" It's a stretch, but who didn't dream big before they became successful?

## THE LAST SECRET

I love you all, even though I don't know you. It's a blessing that I can help you by doing what I most desire and possess the greatest passion for—writing. I have always wanted to be a published author. If you know me, you know that I pursue things until I've driven myself to the cliff of insanity. I'd say that there's no looking back, but I am starting to give myself enough grace to amuse myself with the past, especially the parts of it that catapulted me into my 'right now' and the parts that make me ask, "what if?" It's what gives me a story to tell—distinct from the average 'how to.' I called this book a 'survival guide,' not so much because I wanted to teach you how to do your job—you'll learn that with or without me. Instead, I wanted to share how your frame of thinking can make or break key things in your personal and professional life. My experiences in this field thus far have ranged from pure exhilaration—even mania—to downright breaking my heart. I have shed many good and bad tears on my way to this paragraph, and I believe I'm nowhere near done yet.

I've never been so committed to anything else as I am to pursuing this field, writing, traveling, and most of all—loving myself in each of those activities. The best thing I've learned is that I am not trapped in a box; only that I was trapped in a state of mind. I can, in fact, do my favorite things simultaneously as a result of vetting my one thing first, asking questions endlessly, and faithfully relying on the answers to come. I'm almost just as new here as you are, and for what my idea of the pinnacle of 'success' is... I haven't even touched the hem of the garment. I learned to carry myself like someone who's successful anyway, because I am worthy of it. You too, are worthy of a career that sets you on fire. So pursue it with every bit of your being. With that, you'll not only survive the skilled nursing facility, you'll conquer it.

**CHAPTER FOOTNOTES**

[1]Keller, Gary, and Jay Papasan. 2012. The one thing: the surprisingly simple truth behind extraordinary results. Austin, Tex: Bard Press.

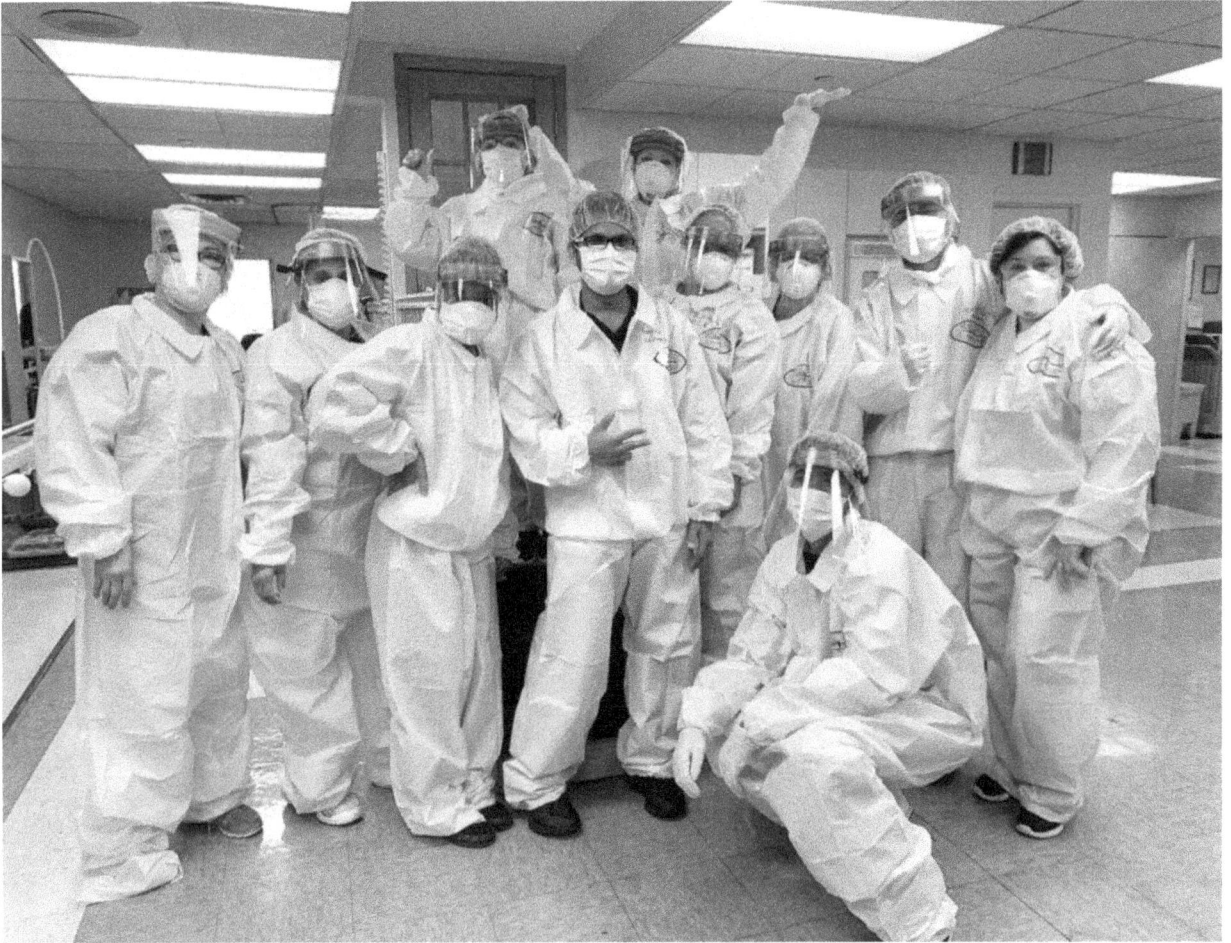

# ACKNOWLEDGEMENTS

I want to be transparent: I struggled with sharing the fact that I was writing this book, because I feared I'd not be taken seriously or seen as someone who doesn't take her job seriously. Generally, I make an extra effort to not stir too many feathers, and I keep a lot to myself. Sharing my experience in this format has been my proudest moment.

I am faithful, and I always thank God first. I thank my family, who was patient as I hogged all the computer time in the last months of writing, and for supporting me financially and spiritually to see me through the end of this project. I thank my mentor, Tasanyia Sebro, and my CFY supervisor, Anna Broniek. I thank my rehab director Michele Petherick and chief clinical dietician Judith Batashoff, who will have an everlasting impact on my journey as an SLP, and probably don't even know it. I thank my friends who are not speech pathologists, but took the time to review my book and other items related to this project.

I take it for no small instance that each of these people were a part of my life, and am grateful for their help somewhere along the way.

# ABOUT THE AUTHOR

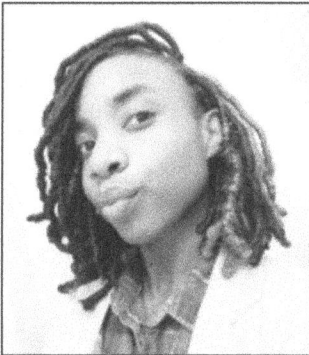

Suleika Pryce is a licensed and certified speech-language pathologist based in Brooklyn, New York. She is a proud alumna of Temple University and received her Master of Science in Speech-Language Pathology from Adelphi University. Suleika has provided intervention for a wide range of populations. Her most advanced practice has been in geriatrics and adult neurological disorders. She primarily treated dysphagia and acquired speech and language disorders in the skilled nursing facility. Most recently, she has transitioned into early intervention and adult in-patient behavioral health.

Tattletales of a Speech-Language Pathologist, the book, is Suleika's inaugural work into authorship, and represents one of her greatest accomplishments. Suleika is also a poetry and fiction writer, and she enjoys teaching literacy and creative expression to school-aged children. She also has an affinity for adults with developmental disabilities and residual effects of traumatic brain injury.

Suleika has founded the organization Tattletales of a Speech-Language Pathologist, which is a community-based initiative to improve partnership and networking of rehabilitative health service providers, especially speech-language pathologists. She coined "good gossip" to reframe people's ideas of the virtue in and need to talk about their experiences in the health field in order to improve them.

"Things. Take. Time. Inevitably. Uncomfortably. You don't always have full control, and when you do, you lose out on the opportunity to take what someone else has to offer to your process."

# Tattletales of a SPEECH-LANGUAGE PATHOLOGIST

## The CFY's Guide To Surviving The Skilled Nursing Facility.

# THANK YOU
## for reading

Feel free to visit www.mytattletalesspeech.com to leave your review, donate, or collect additional resources for the speech-language pathologist.

Also, please take a moment to share your honest opinion. Visit Amazon.com, search for "Tattletales by Suleika Pryce," and click on the "Write a customer review" button. Alternatively, you can leave a review on your favorite review platform.

www.ingramcontent.com/pod-product-compliance
Lightning Source LLC
Chambersburg PA
CBHW081150270326
41930CB00014B/3099